Step by Step®

Management of Clubfoot by Ponseti Technique

Step by Step®
Management of Clubfoot by Ponseti Technique

Second Edition

RA Agrawal
MS(Orthopaedics) AO/ASIF(Germany, Austria) Ilizarov(Russia)
Director
Agrawal Orthopaedic Hospital
Gorakhpur, Uttar Pradesh, India
Past President, ASAMI India

Sureshwar Pandey
MS(Surgery, Orthopaedic) FICS FIAMS FAC FAS FACS FNAMS
Ex-Head and Emeritus Professor
Department of Orthopaedics
RMCH
Ranchi, Jharkhand, India
Emeritus President, Indian Foot and Ankle Society

Rajat Agrawal
MS(Orthopaedics)
Senior Orthopaedic Surgeon
Agrawal Orthopaedic Hospital
Gorakhpur, Uttar Pradesh, India
President, ASAMI India (2023–2025)

JAYPEE BROTHERS MEDICAL PUBLISHERS
The Health Sciences Publisher
New Delhi | London

Jaypee Brothers Medical Publishers (P) Ltd

Headquarters
EMCA House
23/23-B, Ansari Road, Daryaganj
New Delhi 110 002, India
Landline: +91-11-23272143, +91-11-23272703
+91-11-23282021, +91-11-23245672
E-mail: jaypee@jaypeebrothers.com

Corporate Office
Jaypee Brothers Medical Publishers (P) Ltd.
4838/24, Ansari Road, Daryaganj
New Delhi 110 002, India
Phone: +91-11-43574357
Fax: +91-11-43574314
E-mail: jaypee@jaypeebrothers.com

Overseas Office
JP Medical Ltd.
83, Victoria Street, London
SW1H 0HW (UK)
Phone: +44-20 3170 8910
Fax: +44(0)20 3008 6180
E-mail: info@jpmedpub.com

Website: www.jaypeebrothers.com
Website: www.jaypeedigital.com

Inquiries for bulk sales may be solicited at: jaypee@jaypeebrothers.com

***Step by Step®: Management of Clubfoot by Ponseti Technique* / RA Agrawal, Sureshwar Pandey, Rajat Agrawal**

First Edition: 2007

Second Edition: **2025**

ISBN: 978-93-6616-444-1

Printed at: Samrat Offset Pvt. Ltd.

Preface to the Second Edition

Idiopathic clubfoot is perhaps the most common congenital deformity involving the osteoarticular system in a human being. Although the affected person manages to carry out his/her activities of daily living, even the activities for earning the livelihood, as well as any workplace activities, the demands about lasting full correction of foot deformity always hover and haunt him/her. Hence, various conservative or operative or combined efforts have been made to correct the clubfoot deformity. But, truly speaking, none has served the desired purpose, i.e., providing an everlasting, cosmetic, fully functional foot suitable to fit in a normal shoe. However, the Dr Ponseti method of managing the clubfoot *decidedly marks* the starting period in the management of clubfoot.

In late neglected clubfoot deformity, the role of the Ilizarov method has been proved to be useful. If the Ilizarov method is combined with the Ponseti concept of managing the clubfoot, especially in the neglected ones, it will have advantages of both the techniques. We published the first edition of the book in 2007, which was liked by many. Encouraged by the feedback for the first edition, we felt motivated to bring about this second edition. We will be thankful for your fruitful and valuable comments for further improvement.

Through this handbook, we are trying to communicate the master's instructions in our own way for managing the clubfoot in different age groups. Perhaps Dr Ponseti's concentrations has been mainly on managing the neonate clubfoot or clubfoot in early infancy. But the place where we work, as well as in all developing countries, few neonates with clubfoot are brought in for management; rather neglected clubfoot is encountered more frequently. We have attempted to categorize the management age-wise and have suggested how to take advantage of the Ilizarov ring fixator as and when required. Of course, the Ponseti principle has been mostly adhered to.

If a young surgeon, who desires to manage clubfoot especially by the Ponseti technique, derives any help from this handbook, we will be satisfied. We are aware that there may be shortcomings in our book, which we will try to correct with the help of your useful comments and suggestions.

Let us communicate frankly that our aim in producing this monograph is to induct the well-established principle of Ponseti technique of correction of clubfoot through Ilizarov instrumentations principally in the neglected clubfoot.

In preparing this monograph, we have consulted many books and journals and derived ideas and inspiration from several sources. We have tried to acknowledge as and where needed, and also put them as reference. However, we beg apology for any omissions.

Dr John E Herzenberg MD, FRCS has contributed a useful chapter "Tibialis Anterior Transfer in Clubfoot" in this handbook. We are thankful to him. We are also thankful to Global-HELP Publication, who have given us the permission to use and provided original photographs for this book.

We acknowledge the constant help of our sincere colleagues and friends like Mr Munir Ahmad, Mr Anoop, Mr Abhay Mishra, and Dr Shahi.

We are highly thankful to the young and enthusiastic orthopedic surgeon Dr Ashish Agrahari whose dedication and hard work have made the writing of this book possible.

The typing, aligning the manuscript, and improving the script comprise the real tough job in preparing any book and all of that have been done tirelessly with devotion by Ms Smita Dubey who remained alert and active for this work all the time.

The authors could not have concentrated on the work unless the family members had provided them full cooperation. And to this, the dear family of Dr RA Agrawal has stood the test of time, accepting all the eccentricities during the preparation of this book. The contribution of Dr RA Agrawal's wife Mrs Rashmi and daughter Mrs Richa, a software engineer, simply deserve all credits in uninterrupted production of this book.

No book can see the light of the day without the whole-hearted cooperation from the publisher. To this end, we are lucky to have Shri Jitendar P Vij (Group Chairman) and his devoted team who have been with us all the time whenever we needed them. Our sincere thanks go to them.

RA Agrawal
Sureshwar Pandey
Rajat Agrawal

Preface to the First Edition

Clubfoot is being managed for centuries with variable results. There are certain facts about the clubfoot, which have to be acknowledged. The proper etiology of clubfoot is unknown, understanding of the pathoanatomy is unclear and a proper useful classification is yet to be chartered. This is also a fact that most of the orthopaedic surgeons have treated clubfoot and perhaps each one evolved his own mode of management, of course, basic techniques do remain more or less the same.

Management of clubfoot has been mainly on two fronts—non-operative and operative. The consensus has been to start treating clubfoot non-operatively except in unusual circumstances. Non-operative management has been done principally by manipulation and plaster casts. Of the various techniques, that of Hiram Kite remained more or less the accepted procedure with or without some individual variation. However, with the advent of Ponseti technique of cast correction, there appears to be a gradual shift from Kite to Ponseti technique. No technique can yield proper desired results unless the master's instructions are followed to the point. After Ponseti's own publication and publication from Global-HELP organization; perhaps no authentic manual has been published on Ponseti technique.

Through this handbook, we are trying to communicate the master's instructions in our own way for managing the clubfoot in different age groups. Perhaps Dr Ponseti's concentrations have been mainly over managing the neonate clubfoot or clubfoot in early infancy. But the place where we work, as well as in all developing countries, few neonates with clubfoot are brought for management, rather neglected clubfoot is encountered more frequently. We have attempted to categorize the management age-wise and we have suggested for taking advantage of the Ilizarov ring fixator as and when required. Of course, the Ponseti principle has been mostly adhered to.

If the young surgeon, who desires to manage clubfoot especially by Ponseti technique, derives any help from this manual, we will be satisfied. We are aware that there may be shortcomings in our book, which we will try to correct on your useful comments and suggestion.

Let us communicate frankly that our aim in producing this monograph is to induct the well established principle of Ponseti technique of correction of clubfoot through Ilizarov instrumentations principally in the neglected clubfoot.

In preparing this monograph we have consulted many books and journals, derived ideas and inspiration from several sources. We have tried to acknowledge as and where needed, and also put them as reference. However, we beg apology for any ommissions. Dr John E. Herzenberg, MD, FRCS, has contributed a useful chapter on "Tibialis Anterior Transfer in Clubfoot" in this manual. We are thankful to him. We are also thankful to Global-HELP Publication, who have given us the permission to use and provided original photograph for this book.

We acknowledge the constant help of our sincere colleagues and friends like Dr RC Srivasatava, Dr KN Mishra, Dr Pradeep, Mr Arun, Mr Munir Ahmad, Mr Anoop, Ms Harshita, Mr Santosh (Artist) and Mr Shankar Joshi.

We are highly thankful to young and enthusiastic orthopaedic surgeon Dr DP Yadav whose dedication and hard work has made the writing of this book possible.

We are thankful to Dr Rajat Agrawal, the young keen orthopaedic surgeon who laboured hard to provide proper shape of the chapters and the book as a whole.

The typing, aligning the manuscript and improving the script is the real tough job in preparing any book—and all that have been done tirelessly with devotion by Mr Shyam Ji Srivastava who remained alert and active for this work all the time.

The authors could not have concentrated on the work unless the family members would have provided them full cooperation. And to this, the dear family of Dr RA Agrawal has stood the test of time accepting all the eccentricities during the preparation of this book. The contribution of Dr RA Agrawal's wife Mrs Rashmi and daughter Mrs Richa, a software engineer, simply deserve all credits in uninterrupted production of this book.

No book can see the light of the day without whole hearted cooperation from the publisher. To this end we are lucky to have Shri JP Vij (CMD), Mr Tarun Duneja, (GM Publishing) and his devoted team to be with us all the time whenever we needed them. Our whole hearted thanks go to them.

RA Agrawal
Sureshwar Pandey

A Word About Dr Ponseti

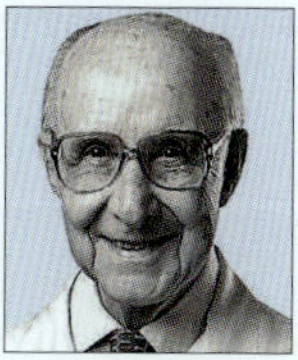

Dr Ignacio V Ponseti, a native of Spain, graduated from the University of Barcelona's medical school in 1936. One day after the Spanish Civil War began, he immediately volunteered with the Government's Republic Army, for treating hundreds of wounded soldiers during the Spanish Civil War. He fled to France after the war and landed in Mexico where he worked as a general practitioner. He arrived in Iowa City in 1941. In 1944, Dr Ponseti joined the faculty of orthopedic surgery at the University of Iowa and retired as Professor Emeritus.

Dr Ponseti took special interest in children with clubfoot and started a new form of manipulative treatment of the congenital clubfoot in 1948 at the University of Iowa Hospitals. This treatment was supported by limited operative interventions based on a clear understanding of the functional anatomy of the foot.

This method yielded optimal results in a high percentage of patients. The study was conducted with a follow-up period of 25–42 years. He published his first paper in 1963. In 1996, the Oxford University Press published his book "Congenital Clubfoot: Fundamentals of Treatment" which confirmed the success of his approach.

The "Ponseti Method" uses manipulations and castings as opposed to the established practice of surgically correcting clubfoot.

Earlier only a handful of orthopedic surgeons used his relatively simple method, but in recent years the pendulum has begun to swing as public and professional awareness has grown. Today, more and more orthopedic surgeons worldwide are recognizing the "Ponseti Method" as the proper and safe way to correct the deformity of clubfoot.

A Subspecialty Orthopaedic Clinic that serves infants with clubfoot at University of Iowa Hospital and Clinics has been named in honor of Dr Ponseti.

Today, even at the age of around 90 years, he still works as a young doctor. Since he developed his nonsurgical treatment for clubfoot 50 years ago, Dr Ponseti has to his credit treatment of more than 2,000 children. He has devoted his life to the service of children.

He is internationally known for his clubfoot treatment that is known today as the "Ponseti Method."

Contents

CHAPTER 1

Introduction

The high incidence of clubfoot makes it a common congenital deformity. Clubfoot has been derived from the word **club** meaning a heavy tapering stick with knobby end. Worldwide incidence is about one to two per thousand live births with higher incidence reported in Maori, Polynesians and Hawaiians. The ratio of male to female is 3:1 and around 40% cases are bilateral.

The earliest evidence of clubfoot dates back to the Egyptian period and drawing of clubfoot has been found on the walls of tombs, a statue of distrophic dwarf with clubfoot is among the collections of Tutankhamen.

The archeological experts of Mexico have reported that Azetecs knew about clubfoot and treated it with splints made from cactus leaves. The Indian surgeon Sushruta 500 BC recommended correction of such deformity by massage in infancy, splinting in early childhood and adaptive foot-wear in adults. It is mentioned in *Corpus Hippocrates* that gentle repeated manipulation could effectively correct the clubfoot deformity, this basic principle still holds well.

Earliest account of surgical intervention for correction was subcutaneous tendo-Achilles tenotomy performed by

Lorenz in Frankford in 1782. Talectomy was first performed by Lund in 1872. With the modern era of orthopedics equipped with superior antisepsis, anaesthesia, tourniquet, etc., evolved, the better operative treatment. Phelp (1890), an orthopaedist from New York, described a single stage medial plantar soft tissue release with lengthening of tendons. He also performed an osteotomy of the neck of talus with wedge resection of calcaneum. During 1900–1930 many surgical methods evolved including correction of clubfoot by soft tissue release at an early age of 3 years by Codvilla from Italy. Few orthopaedists advocated nonsurgical management after poor long-term results of operative treatment.

Thus, the whole century was spent in exploring, planning, and modifying those treatments, which produced unsatisfactory results. This period enhanced the knowledge of pathoanatomy of the clubfoot. In 1866, Adams differentiated congenital clubfoot from acquired clubfoot variety due to neurological and other causes.

Till few years the most accepted method of non-operative treatment of clubfoot was that advocated by Hiram Kite in 1930 through serial manipulation and immobilisation in plaster cast.

Ponseti's Principle

Method of Kite was studied by Ignacio V. Ponseti, who had an opportunity to observe his method in 1960. Ponseti concluded that the method was lengthy and short of satisfactory results. After an extensive study and reviewing, he came to the conclusion that the major flaw of Kite's method was the attempt to correct the components of the deformity one by one instead of simultaneously correcting them. The movements at ankle and subtalar joints are coupled movement and it is almost impossible to reproduce them independently without affecting the other joint. Ponseti studied these movements extensively by dissection and radiocinematography and developed a non-operative method to correct the clubfoot deformity.

Based on his studies he developed and refined a uniform type of treatment schedule in the late forties. In 40 years of his follow-up experience, he found the method optimum. The method is very easy to master and surgery can be avoided by this method. The method requires lesser duration and produces superior results in comparison to extensive manipulation and surgery by other methods. In 1948, he proposed following guidelines for treatment of the clubfoot:

a. All the components of clubfoot deformity should be corrected simultaneously except obviously the equinus, which is finally corrected at the last.
b. The cavus is the result of pronation of forefoot in relation to the hindfoot—it is corrected as the foot is abducted in supinated position of forefoot and thereby placing it in proper alignment with the hindfoot.
c. While the whole foot is held in supination, it is gradually and gently abducted under the talus which is held secured against rotation in the ankle mortise by applying counter-pressure with the thumb over the lateral aspect of the head of the talus.
d. The heel varus and supination of foot will automatically get corrected when the entire foot is fully abducted under the talus. The foot should never be everted.

e. Finally, the equinus is corrected by dorsiflexing the foot. The tendo-Achilles subcutaneous tenotomy may be required to facilitate this correction.

This method is being used by us and has produced better result than previously adopted method for the treatment of clubfoot. Assimilating the principles of the technique, we at our centre implemented this method of gradual manipulation in older neglected cases with the help of Ilizarov ring fixators and are happy to get expected results.

This book is a step toward providing a simplified method along with other information regarding clubfoot deformity so that it can be easily mastered and implemented.

CHAPTER 2

Planes and Biomechanics of Foot

Foot in real sense forms the footing of the human race on the earth. Human foot is considered to be an amazing and complex piece of bioengineering. A number of bones along with multiple joints contribute to its skeletal framework. The talus and the calcaneus together form the hindfoot, the navicular, cuboid and the three cuneiforms form the mid-foot whereas the forefoot is formed by the metatarsals along with the phalanges. The arrangement of the associated joints in the foot is such that the movements at one joint influence the movements at the other joints in such a way that a biomechanical kinetic chain is created that ensures optimal functioning of this unit.

Planes

In any three-dimensional assessment, three planes have to be considered and this holds true for the ankle and foot as well. The three planes are **(Fig. 2.1)**:

1. Sagittal
2. Horizontal
3. Frontal or coronal

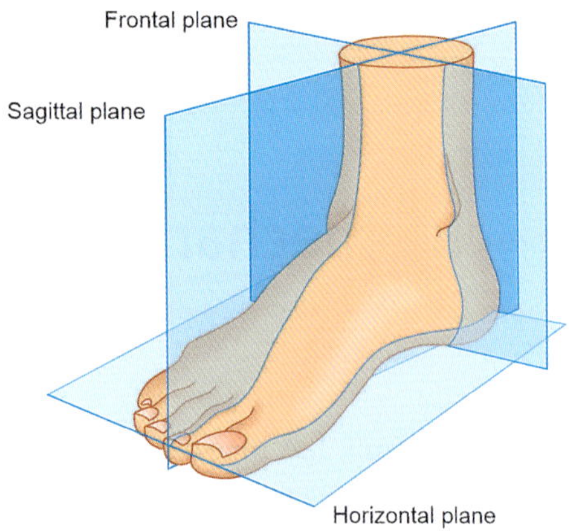

FIG. 2.1: 3-D picture of foot showing planes

While describing any deformity, usually the first two planes are considered. Besides these planes, rotational deformities are assessed against certain axis, which exists separately for each movement.

The Biomechanics and Kinesiology of Ankle Joint

In a human being with bipedal locomotion, the biomechanics of the foot has been oriented to serve the basic and refined functions of the foot. The basic functions of the foot are:

1. To receive the weight of the body
2. To distribute the weight throughout the foot
3. To help in locomotion in bipedal fashion
4. To provide soundless springing gait
5. To execute fine functions like dancing, gymnastic activities etc.

To achieve all the above goals, minimal requirement is the plantigrade foot in which the weight is borne by different parts of the foot in a systematic order. There have been several opinions about the weight distribution in the foot but the most accepted opinion is in the following way. Unit-wise, if the body weight is 24 units, then each foot receives 12 units, of these 12 units 50%, i.e., 6 units are borne by the hindfoot and 6 by the forefoot in which 2 units are borne by the ball of great toe and 1 each for other toes. The midfoot is mainly concerned about dynamic distribution of the weight mainly through the medial longitudinal arch. From hindfoot, the weight is transmitted to the forefoot in a piano-distribution pattern mainly through the transverse arches. Any deviation from this plantigrade pattern will lead to deformity (ies) in the foot.

The ankle joint becomes significant due to its function in load bearing, locomotive and propulsive action. The complex movements of the foot which occur below this joint at subtalar and forefoot joints are important for adaptation according to the ground surface. The foot is the body's primary contact point with the ground and since the ground is often uneven, the foot must be adaptable. In fact, it is reasonable to regard the foot as the foundation upon which everything else stands, and the problems that alter the mechanics of the foot will influence body posture and vertebral structures.

Ankle joint: It consists of two components:

1. *Ankle mortise*: It is formed by the lower end of tibia and fibula attached with inferior interosseous tibiofibular ligament and medial and lateral malleoli.

2. *Talus*: It articulates with ankle mortise through its dome on the superior articular surface and the articular facets on the either side of the body of talus for articulating with the malleoli.

Movements: Ankle joint is basically a uniaxial hinge joint. Though the articular surface of talar dome is saddle shaped to some extent, the main movements are plantar flexion and dorsiflexion. Dorsiflexion is produced mainly by tibialis anterior and peroneus tertius assisted by extensor digitorum longus and extensor hallucis longus. Plantar flexion is produced mainly by gastrocnemius and soleus and is assisted by plantaris, tibialis posterior, flexor hallucis longus and flexor digitorum longus.

Subtalar joint: The components of subtalar joint are the articular surfaces on inferior surface of talus and superior surface of calcaneum.

To understand the motion in clubfoot one has to understand the subtalar joint complex. Subtalar joint is a functional unit formed by the anterior and posterior articulation between talus and calcaneum. The posterior articulation is called talocalcaneal joint while anterior articulation is regarded as part of talocalcaneonavicular joint. Talocalcaneonavicular joint is formed by two joints—the anterior part of subtalar joint and talonavicular joint. Subtalar joint complex consists of talocalcaneal and talocalcaneonavicular joint. The centre of rotation of the subtalar joint is talocalcaneal interosseous ligament, which consists of two bands **(Fig. 2.2A)**. The joint participates in the movement of inversion and eversion of foot. Talocalcaneonavicular articulation has some features of ball and socket joint, the head of talus fits on the socket formed partly by navicular and partly by calcaneum.

Subtalar axis: The subtalar joint is single axis joint, in transverse plane subtalar axis deviates approximately 23° medial to the long axis of the foot, and approximately 42° from the horizontal plane **(Figs 2.2B and C)**.

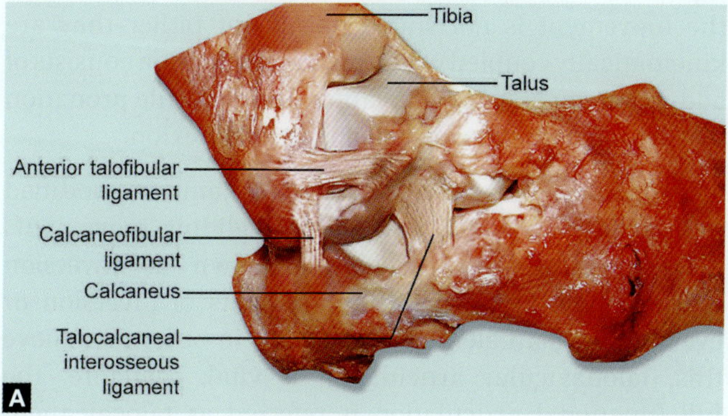

FIG. 2.2A: Photograph showing talocalcaneal interosseous ligament

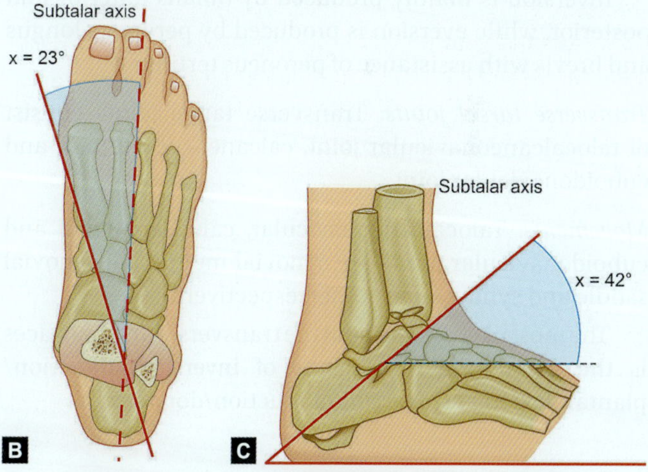

FIGS. 2.2B AND C: Sketch diagram showing subtalar axis

Movements at subtalar joint, i.e., inversion and eversion take place around this oblique axis which runs forward, upward and medially, passing from back of calcaneum, through the sinus tarsi to emerge at the superio-medial aspect of the neck of talus. Due to the obliquity of the axis, the movement is not single movement rather they are kinematically coupled which means, supination consists of adduction, inversion, and plantar flexion; while pronation consists of abduction, eversion, and dorsiflexion.

Movements: Talocalcaneal (subtalar) joint is modified multiaxial joint which permits only gliding movements between talus and calcaneum known as inversion and eversion. However, the movements of inversion or eversion have an element of rotation; in order to achieve this, talonavicular articulation is vital, therefore, the full functional articulation is referred as talocalcaneo-navicular joint, which is thus multiaxial.

Inversion is mainly produced by tibialis anterior and posterior, while eversion is produced by peroneus longus and brevis with assistance of peroneus tertius.

Transverse tarsal joints: Transverse tarsal joints consist of talocalcaneonavicular joint, calcaneocuboid joint and cuboidonavicular joint.

Movements: Talocalcaneonavicular, calcaneocuboid and cuboidonavicular joints are synovial multiaxial, synovial saddle and syndesmotic joints respectively.

The most likely outcome at the transverse tarsal surfaces is the compound movements of inversion/adduction/plantar flexion and eversion/abduction/dorsiflexion.

Tarsometatarsal joints: They are formed by cuneiforms, cuboid and metatarsals.

Movements: Only slight gliding and translation is possible between the individual joint surfaces which permit just a few degrees of dorsiflexion and a little more plantar flexion.

Clubfoot: In clubfoot, kinematics is greatly altered due to severe shortening of medial and posterior tarsal ligaments and tightness of tibialis posterior and gastrosoleus muscles. The fibrotic and contracted deltoid ligament holds the calcaneum in inversion. The navicular is medially displaced and inverted due to fibrosis of tibionavicular ligament, plantar calcaneonavicular ligament (spring ligament) and pull of the tight tibialis posterior tendon. Since the intertarsal joints are interdependent, displacement of the navicular induces medial displacement and inversion of cuboid and calcaneus.

Mobility of the posterior part of foot is severely restricted. Only a few degree of passive abduction can be done in rigid feet, while 20–30° abduction is possible in less severe cases. In spite of displaced and deformed tarsal joints, they are congruent. The joints become incongruent when correction of the deformity is attempted rapidly. Therefore, correction should be done gradually allowing gradual remodelling of the joint surfaces.

CHAPTER 3

Etiology and Pathogenesis

Despite years of pondering to know the actual cause of clubfoot, we are still beating about the bush. Clubfoot may be caused by both extrinsic or environmental and genetic factors.

Etiology

Extrinsic Causes

Congenital clubfoot may be caused by extrinsic or environmental factors without presence of any genetic factor.

It is seen with congenital annular bands but it was also found that clubfoot is secondary to the decreased capacity of uterus resulting from the early rupture of amnion, with the chorion remaining intact.

It has also been found in infants who have survived the mother's attempt to abort with the use of sodium aminopterin.

The use of d-tubocurarine during first trimester of pregnancy is also associated with arthrogryposis and severe talipes equinovarus.

From these examples, it is inferred that numerous causes including a small uterine cavity, intrauterine position at the time of d-tubocurarine paralysis and drugs ingested by the mother can cause congenital clubfoot in absence of any genetic cause.

Genetic Causes

There is a group of children who inherit clubfoot strictly in Mendelian fashion. These children have clubfoot as a part of numerous syndromes.

Autosomal dominant inheritance: Typical example of this inheritance is whistling—face syndrome or craniocarpotarsal dysplasia. If both parents and the child have this syndrome there is one in two chances that each subsequent sibling will also have the syndrome and severe clubfoot.

Autosomal recessive inheritance: Autosomal recessive inheritance of clubfoot is seen in diastrophic dwarfism, which is present with micromelia, joint contracture, scoliosis, thumb deformities and severe clubfoot. One-fourth of subsequent siblings of children with diastrophic dwarfism may be expected. The second example of autosomal recessive inheritance is Larsen's syndrome. It is also seen with Smith–Lemli–Opitz syndrome. Fine et al reported on a child with this syndrome who had severe varus deformity and equinus of hindfoot. Clubfoot may be inherited as a part of X-linked recessive condition. Gorlin et al reported Pierre Robin syndrome with congenital heart malformation and clubfoot.

Cytogenetic abnormalities: Various cytogenetic abnormalities are associated with clubfoot. Clark et al reported on a family with trisomy 6q25 → 6qter in two sisters resulting from maternal 6; 11 translocation. Two affected siblings had severe clubfoot in addition to multiple abnormalities including mental retardation, microcephaly, flattening of occiput, flat nasal bridge, low set ears, micrognathia, dental anomalies, webbed neck, scoliosis, joint contracture and short tapered fingers.

Insley (1967) reported the association of clubfoot with a deficiency of a part of the long arm of chromosome 18. These individuals have micrognathia, carp-like mouth, cryptorchidism, mental retardation and severe bilateral talipes equinovarus.

Thus, syndromes are produced by both excess of cytogenetic material and by deletion of a portion of a chromosome, which in turn can cause severe clubfoot in children.

Multifactorial inheritance: The most common form of congenital clubfoot is the idiopathic variety found in the otherwise normal infant in whom no syndrome, Mendelian disorder, cytogenetic abnormality or extrinsic causes can be found. Therefore, idiopathic variety should be a diagnosis of exclusion.

Palmer altered his view to support a multifactorial system of inheritance. Possibly intrauterine factors have some effect. According to his view, there is a set of genes causing clubfoot that is present in varied amount in individuals. A variation in the distribution of gene frequently exists in the population; some people have substantially more of these genes than the average, and some have substantially fewer. If the number of these genes in a child exceeds, an unidentified threshold value, he or she will be affected with clubfoot. Since boys are affected twice as often as girls, the threshold number of genes is assumed to be lower for boys.

Wynne-Davies concluded that a decreasing incidence of the disorder, as the relationship to the patient becomes more remote, could be indicative of a dominant gene with reduced penetrance or a multifactorial inheritance system.

In conclusion, idiopathic talipes equinovarus is primarily caused by a multifactorial inheritance system. This system is modified by intrauterine environmental factors and possibly is affected by gene acting in a dominant fashion.

Pathogenesis

Hersh (1967) described the presence of a disc like mass of fibrous tissue lying between the medial malleolus and the medial side of the navicular bone. He found that medial malleolus, sustentaculum tali and navicular were bound together by this mass, which consisted of the contracted tibialis posterior tendon, the deltoid and the spring ligaments (Turco 1971).

Fried (1959) in the study of 56 clubfoot patients noted that insertion of tibialis posterior was always thick and like hard fibrous mass at the site of insertion, covering medial side of tarsus.

Zimmy et al (1985) found fibroblastic contracture similar to that of Dupuytren's contracture on electron microscopic study. Therefore, he postulated that myofibroblast like cells were the cause of medial contracture in severe clubfoot.

Kohei et al (1994) studied histomorphometric and immunohistochemical properties of clubfoot in aborted foetuses. Their histomorphometric results indicated that talar deformity was not the primary lesion. Histological and immunohistochemical findings showed that the cells and collagen fibres of the medial ankle ligaments of clubfoot appeared to be the site of the earliest changes, whereby they had lost their spatial orientation and had contracted. In severe clubfoot before the third trimester of gestation, myofibroblast like cells seemed to create a disorder of the ligaments resembling fibromatosis. This led to contraction and resulted in typical clubfoot deformity.

CHAPTER 4

Pathoanatomy

Antonio Scarpa first described pathological anatomy of clubfoot in 1803. He reported the medial and plantar displacement of the navicular, cuboid, and calcaneum around the talus. Displacement of the navicular and calcaneum produces supination of foot. Contracture of the ligaments, joint capsules and tendons maintain this pathological malalignment of joints, described as equinovarus.

Bones

Talus is deformed in such a way that anterior end is deviated medially and plantarward. Neck of talus is short and projects medially, the body is smaller and malplaced in ankle mortice. The talar-neck-body declination angle is invariably decreased with the neck axis approximating 90° to the axis of body in some specimens, compared to the normal 150° to 160°. The articular surface of the talar head is found so close to the body that a true neck is not present.

Navicular is flattened, medially displaced, adducted and inverted. Medial tuberosity is enlarged with wide area for insertion of enlarged tibialis posterior tendon.

Body of *calcaneum* is flexed with medial bow. Its length is either normal or longer than the calcaneum of normal controls. It is adducted and inverted beneath the talus, therefore, most of the anterior tuberosity of calcaneum is under the head of talus and is not palpable. The longitudinal axes of calcaneum and talus become almost parallel.

Cuboid is medially displaced and inverted. Only medial part of anterior tuberosity of calcaneum articulates with cuboid.

Cuneiforms and metatarsals are adducted but they remain normal in shape.

The foot of a 3 days old still born infant having clubfoot deformity was dissected and it was found that navicular is medially displaced and articulates only with the medial aspect of the head of the talus. The cuneiforms are seen to be on the right of the navicular, and the cuboid is underneath it. The calcaneocuboid joint is directed posteromedially. The anterior two thirds of the calcaneum is seen underneath the talus. The tendons of the tibialis anterior, extensor hallucis longus, and extensor digitorum longus are medially displaced **(Fig. 4.1)**.

Joints, Capsules and Ligaments

Talocalcaneal articulation is disturbed significantly. Anterior joint is very narrow or absent, whereas the middle varies in size. Posterior joint is short with lateral inclination.

Some of the ligaments and capsules of affected joints become adapted to the altered joints and their positions because they are either folded or stretched, whereas other ligaments are greatly shortened and thickened. Anterior part of deltoid ligament and plantar calcaneo-navicular ligaments are short and thick. Medial talocalcaneal ligament is markedly thickened **(Fig. 4.2A)**. In many cases they are distorted and matted together with the adjoining

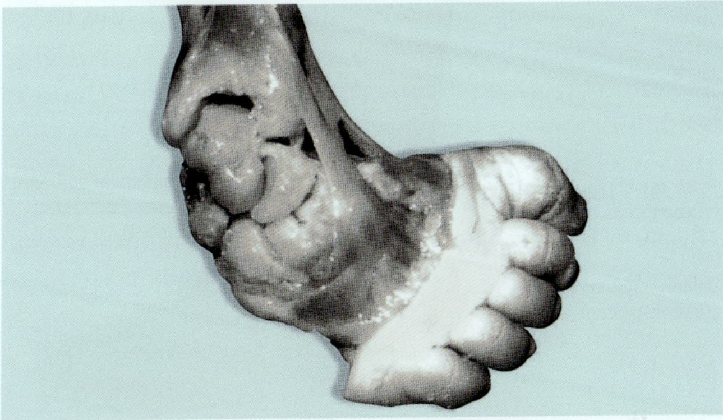

FIG. 4.1: Dissection of a 3-day-old infant's foot showing pathological anatomy of clubfoot

Courtesy: Global-HELP Organization 2003

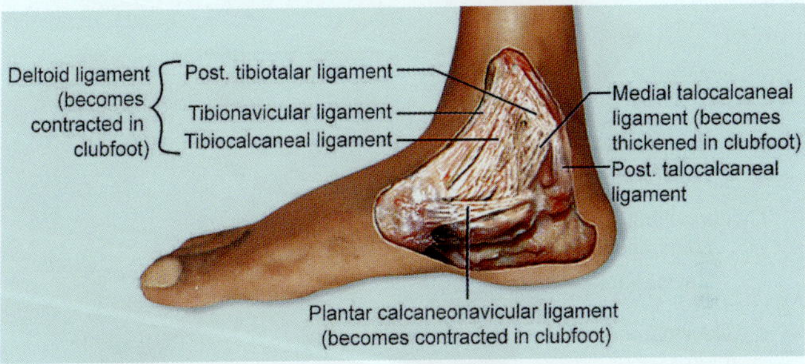

FIG. 4.2A: Photograph showing normal ligaments of ankle and foot from medial side

tendon sheaths. The posterior tibiotalar, anterior and posterior talofibular and calcaneofibular ligaments are also thick and short **(Fig. 4.2B)**.

The interosseous talocalcaneal ligaments in sinus tarsi are under-developed **(Fig. 4.2C)**.

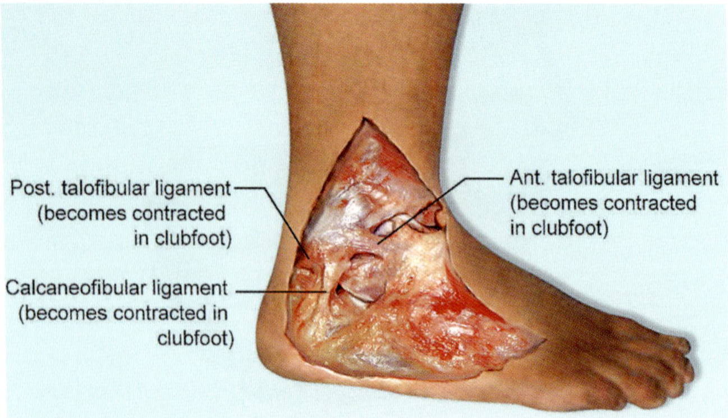

FIG. 4.2B: Photograph showing normal ligaments of ankle and foot from lateral side

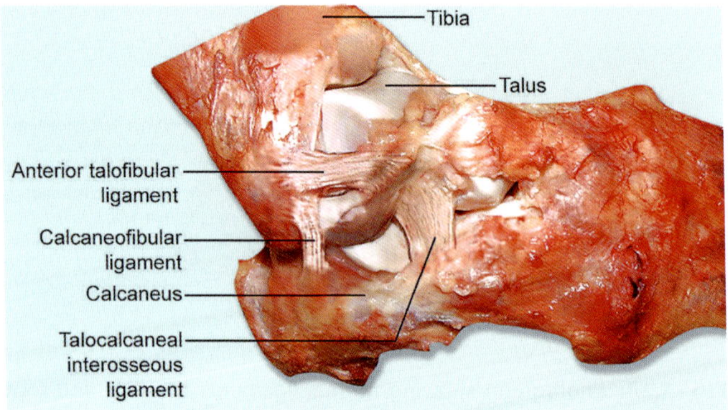

FIG. 4.2C: Photograph showing normal ligaments of foot from lateral side

The bifurcate ligament is stretched and thin. The calcaneocuboid ligament and navicular cuneiform ligaments are normal or slightly enlarged. The plantar fascia is thick and contracted **(Fig. 4.2D)**.

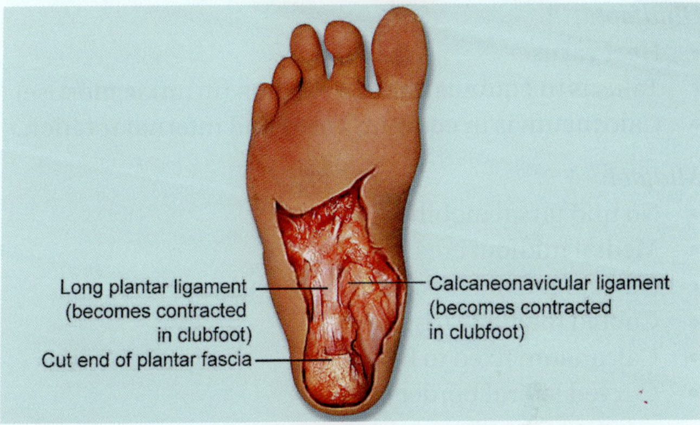

FIG. 4.2D: Photograph showing ligaments of foot from plantar side

Muscles and Tendons

Muscle tendon units of gastrosoleus and tibialis posterior are smaller and shorter **(Fig. 4.3B)**. The distal part of tibialis posterior tendon is increased two to three times in size and its sheath is thickened and matted to the ligaments on the medial aspect of foot. Insertion of tendo-Achilles is slightly medial on the posterior calcaneal tuberosity.

Pathological anatomy can be summarised as:

Gross:

- Affected limb may be shortened
- Calf muscle is atrophic and foot is short
- Medial rotation of tibia.

Joints:

- Ankle and subtalar joints are in fixed equinus
- Posterior displacement of lateral malleolus.

Hindfoot:
- Heel varus
- Talus is in equinus, medial rotation (in ankle mortise)
- Calcaneum is in equinus, varus and internal rotation.

Midfoot:
- No mid tarsal mobility
- Medial midfoot crease
- Navicular fixed to medial malleolus
- Cuboid medially displaced
- Calcaneum fixed to fibula
- Curved lateral border of foot.

Forefoot:
- Forefoot pronated
- Depressed first metatarsal.

Tendons:

Contracture of tendons and soft tissues **(Figs 4.3A to C)**:
- Tendo-Achilles
- Tibialis posterior
- Long toe flexor
- Tibialis anterior
- Extensor digitorum longus
- Extensor hallucis longus
- Plantar aponeurosis
- Abductor hallucis
- Flexor digitorum brevis (causes cavus of foot).

Ligaments

Contracture of ligaments:
- Spring ligament
- Deltoid ligament
- Calcaneofibular ligament

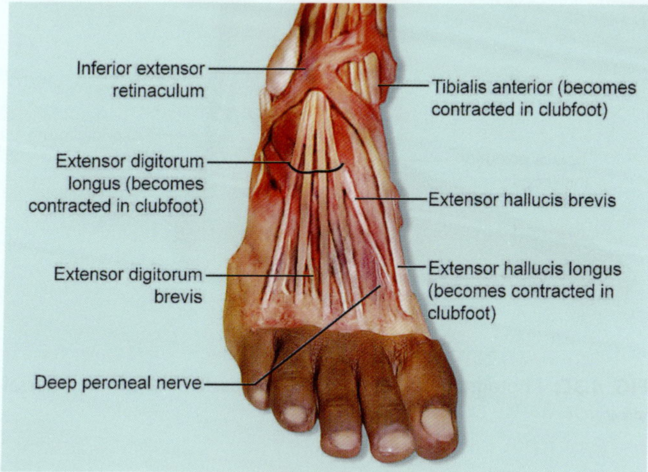

FIG. 4.3A: Photograph showing involved muscle in clubfoot in anterior view

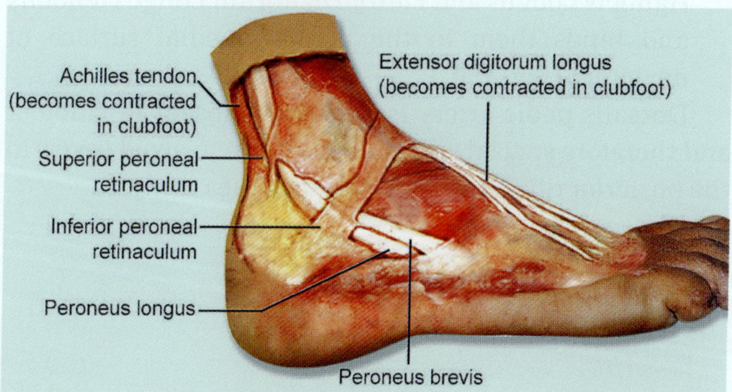

FIG. 4.3B: Photograph showing involved muscle in clubfoot in medial view

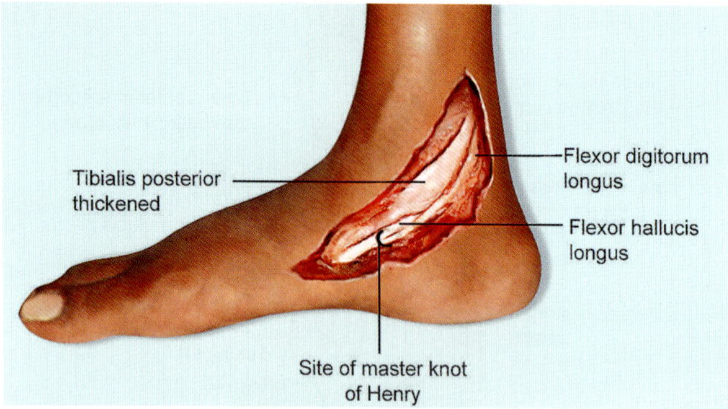

FIG. 4.3C: Photograph showing involved muscle in clubfoot in dorsal view

- Talofibular ligament
- Contracture of Master Knot of Henry: Master knot of Henry is the fibrous slip that envelops the Flexor Hallucis Longus and Flexor Digitorum Longus tendons and binds them to the plantar medial surface of navicular **(Fig. 4.3C)**.

Dorsalis pedis artery is frequently absent in clubfoot and therefore special care must be taken to avoid injury to the posterior tibial artery during surgeries.

CHAPTER 5

Clinical History and Examination

The family history to detect any congenital deformity in parents and past history of the child should be taken, especially about previous treatment. Advancement and widespread use of ultrasonography during pregnancy has greatly increased the chances of diagnosis of deformities. Clubfoot can be diagnosed at a mean gestational age of 22.1 weeks. This helps the expectant parents to decide upon the continuation of pregnancy and cope with the deformity postnatally **(Fig. 5.1)**.

The child should be fully undressed during examination and it should be carried out in supine position followed by prone position to check any possible anomaly on head, neck, chest, trunk and spine. A thorough neurological examination should never be ignored to detect any hidden spinal abnormality. Examination of joints, especially for range of motion and stiffness, is of utmost importance due to congenital disorder like arthrogryposis multiple congenita, which carries a bad prognosis. Treatment plan will vary according to stiffness of joint and in some cases it may require early surgery.

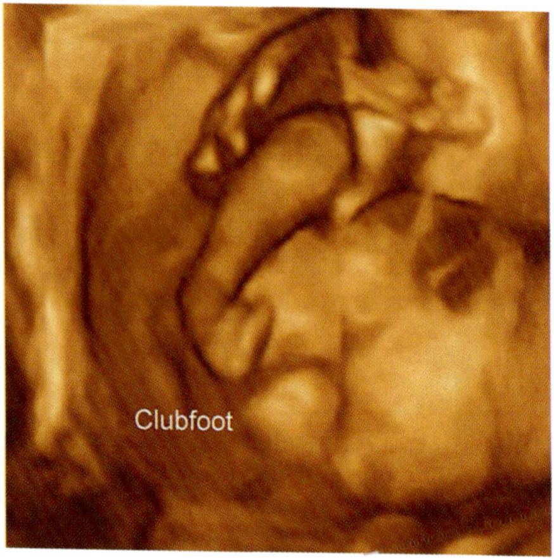

FIG. 5.1: Ultrasonogram showing clubfoot in 20 weeks foetus
Courtesy: Bhola Hospital, Kurukshetra

Foot should be examined in sagittal plane from medial side for equinus deformity, in horizontal plane from top for rotation around talus, from plantar side for adduction deformity and in frontal plane (from back) for varus deformity.

The length of both extremities and circumference of thigh and calf should be measured to see proper development of musculature. The skin folds of thigh, ankle and foot should be recorded along with degree of equinus, heel varus and forefoot adduction, cavus and foot supination.

Varying degrees of severity and rigidity can be encountered at the first examination. Three landmarks should be noted—the position of malleoli in relation to tibial crest and tuberosity to visualise tibial torsion, the head of talus to see displacement of navicular around it and calcaneal tuberosity for its development and varus deformity.

If conservative treatment was undertaken, it is essential to know how many serial plaster casts were applied and which technique was adopted. It is also essential to know what were the factors due to which deformities could not be corrected and why the recurrence took place, the knowledge of all these factors is essential before starting the treatment.

One should not confuse adduction of clubfoot with metatarsus adductus deformity as it is an isolated deformity where heel does not go in varus instead it may show moderate to severe valgus **(Figs 5.2A to D)**. Apart from this, equinus deformity is not found with metatarsus adductus, which is a feature of clubfoot.

Examination of Foot

While examining the foot the surgeon/clinician should hold toes and metatarsals with one hand while with other hand both malleoli are felt from front with thumb on lateral malleolus and index finger on medial malleolus **(Fig. 5.3)**.

Lateral malleolus is more prominent than medial malleolus. Medial malleolus is less prominent because the navicular is shifted towards medial malleolus hiding its tip. On sliding the index finger and thumb downward, the thumb comes on prominent head of talus while the index finger rests on the top of navicular. With the hand holding the toes and metatarsals, the foot is abducted while index finger of the other hand pushes the navicular downward and laterally **(Fig. 5.4)**. Motion and position of navicular in

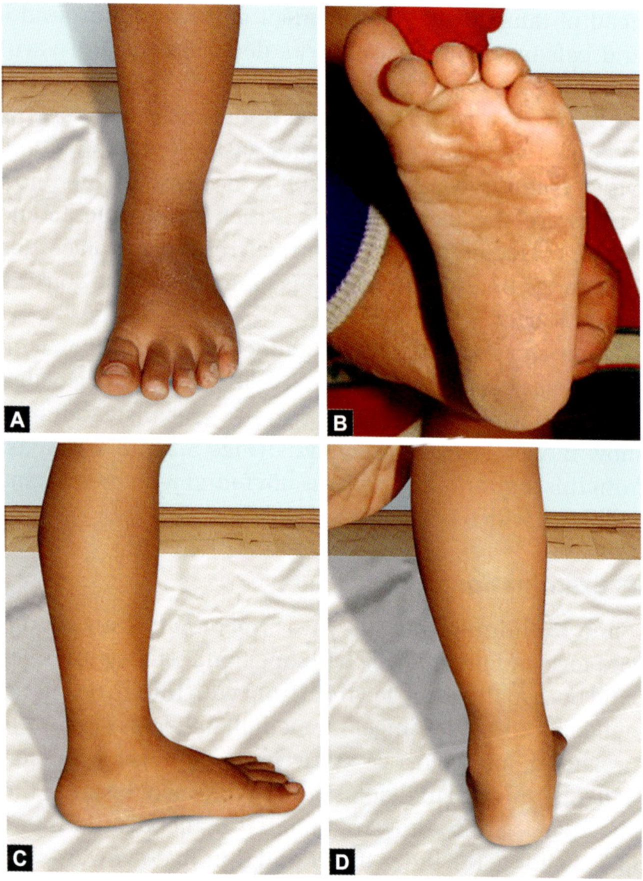

FIGS. 5.2A TO D: Photographs showing metatarsus adductus deformity without any heel varus or equinus deformity

relation to medial malleolus will determine the stiffness of foot. On the lateral side, head of the talus can be palpated with thumb.

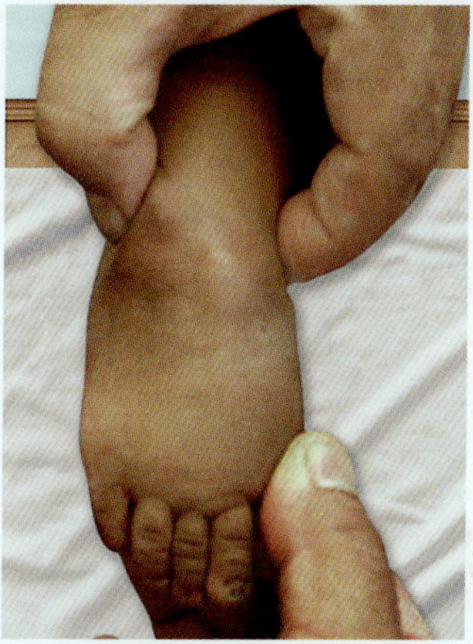

FIG. 5.3: Method of examination: Hold the toes and metatarsals with one hand and feel the malleoli from the front with the thumb and the index finger of the other hand

Calcaneocuboid joint can be palpated easily to know the position of cuboid and its displacement. As there is loosening of ligaments between navicular and cuboid, abduction of forefoot will bring cuboid from medially displaced position to normal along with navicular.

Palpation of cuneiforms is done in front of navicular. First metatarsal is identified in equinus position. In young children first metatarsal can be dorsiflexed as plantar fascia is not so tight but in older children it is difficult to dorsiflex it due to tightness of plantar fascia.

Severity of the clubfoot can be determined by:

1. Congenital atrophy (but tight) due to contracture of calf muscles
2. Degree of equinus
3. Varus of heel

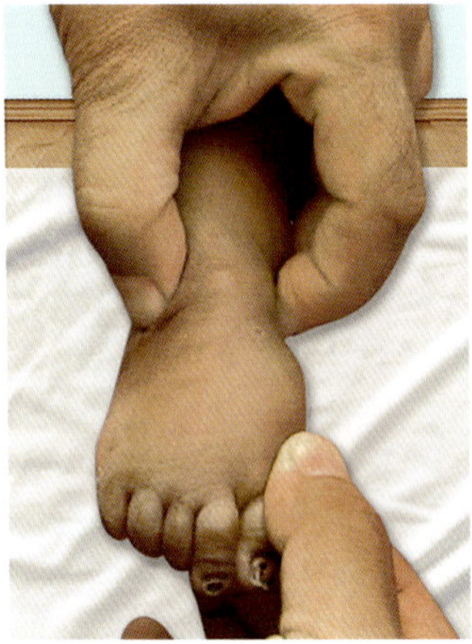

FIG. 5.4: Method of examination: Slide the thumb and index finger downward to feel the head of talus and navicular. Hold the toes and metatarsals with the other hand and feel the movement of the navicular. The distance between the medial malleolus and the navicular is measured which suggests the degree of displacement of the navicular

4. Rigidness of adduction of forefoot
5. Medial displacement of navicular
6. Depth of skin creases on posterior aspect of ankle and medial aspect of foot

By measuring the distance between medial malleolus and navicular one can assess severity of clubfoot clinically. Thus, the role of thorough clinical history and examination can never be omitted.

CHAPTER 6

Photography and Radiological Evaluation

Photography

Keeping the record of cases is core for assessment of deformity correction. It should be done in every case before treatment and in every follow-up.

Photographs should be taken for equinus deformity from medial side **(Fig. 6.1A)**, for varus/valgus deformity from the back **(Fig. 6.1B)**, for midfoot rotation from the top **(Fig. 6.1C)** and for forefoot adduction on hindfoot from plantar side **(Fig. 6.1D)**.

Radiological Evaluation

Radiological evaluation is necessary to assess the deviated position and interrelationship of bones of the foot, any associated bony or joint problems and radiological measurement of different angles.

Anteroposterior standing view with 24° cephalad angulation and lateral standing view should be taken. The main angle visible in lateral view is talocalcaneal and in anteroposterior view is talocalcaneal, talo-first metatarsal and calcaneo-fifth metatarsal.

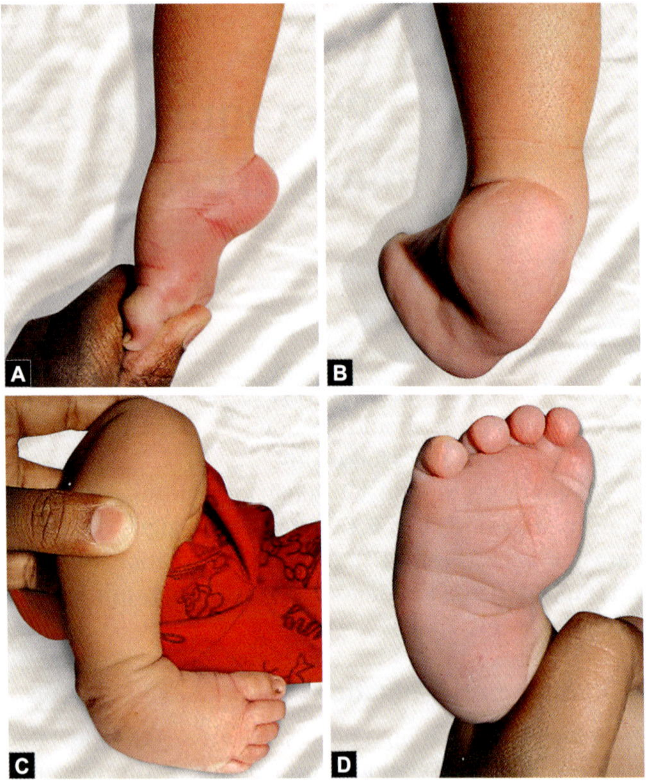

FIGS 6.1A TO D: From medial side for equinus deformity, from back for heel varus, from top for midfoot rotation, from plantar side for forefoot adduction on hindfoot

Radiographs are not very helpful while assessing the deformity as ossification occurs late in children but it may be helpful in cases of recurrence and in older children to plan the line of management.

It is difficult to estimate the accurate position of tarsal bones in roentgenograms of infants, because the centre of ossification of the three visible tarsal bones (calcaneum, talus, and cuboid) is small, oblong, and eccentrically positioned. The navicular, the most displaced component of this deformity, does not ossify until the age of 3–4 years. The views of Rose et al (1985), who studied the flat foot in the child—'radiographs are not helpful, being flat images of a three-dimensional situation', are fully agreed upon. Diagnostic lines and angle change if viewed in a different axis. In addition, the ossific centres for all the foot bones can be drawn accurately only after the age of 6 years. Cummings et al (1994) express similar concern about the reliability of angle measurements of infants' feet. Furthermore, in our experience with long-term results, the talocalcaneal angle does not accurately predict the success or failure of treatment.

Talocalcaneal angle: The talocalcaneal angle is the angle subtended between a line through long axis of talus and another line through long axis of calcaneus. Angle should be calculated in both anteroposterior and lateral view **(Fig. 6.2A)**.

Talocalcaneal index: It represents the sum of talocalcaneal angle in both anteroposterior and lateral view. Talocalcaneal index in clubfoot ranges from 16° to 51° (mean 37.7°); in the normal feet from 37° to 64° (mean 52.3°).

Foot alignment: The alignment of forefoot in relation with the hindfoot is evaluated in anteroposterior view on both medial and lateral aspect of the foot with the help of talar first metatarsal and calcaneal fifth metatarsal angles.

Talocalcaneal angle	**Clubfoot**		**Normal foot**	
	Angle (Degree)	**Mean (Degree)**	**Angle (Degree)**	**Mean (Degree)**
AP view	4–25	15.7	13–29	20.7
Lat. view	10–34	23.1	17–46	31.6
Talocalcaneal angle (as seen in anteroposterior roentgenogram)	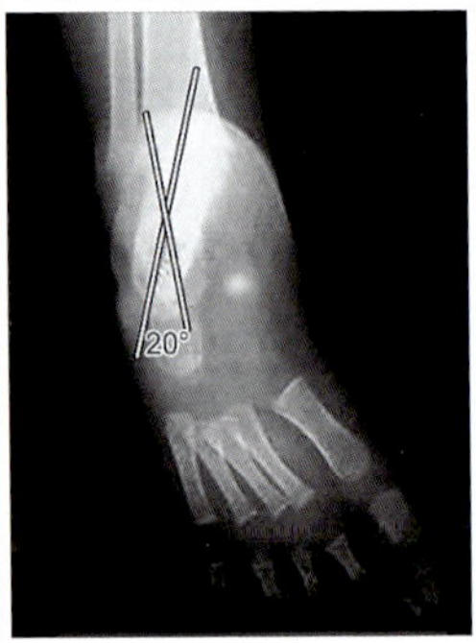 **Clubfoot**		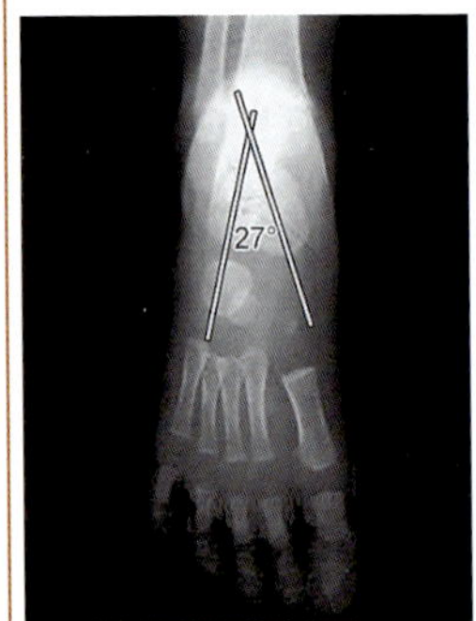 **Normal foot**	
Talocalcaneal angle (as seen in lateral roentgenogram)	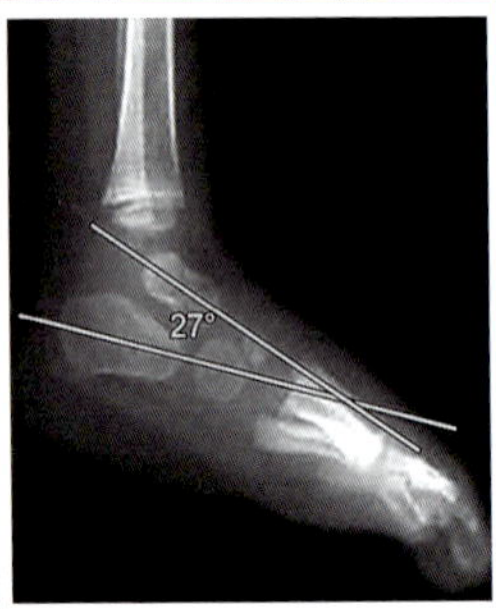 **Clubfoot**		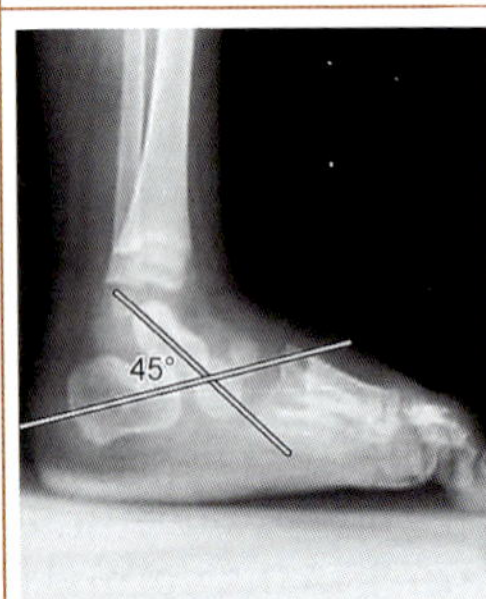 **Normal foot**	

FIG. 6.2A: Talocalcaneal angle in clubfoot and normal foot with radiographs (Ponseti et al 1981)

	Clubfoot		Normal foot	
	Angle (Degree)	**Mean (Degree)**	**Angle (Degree)**	**Mean (Degree)**
Talar first metatarsal	–10 to +33	+3.28	–20 to +11	–3.37
calcaneal fifth metatarsal	–20 to +20	–4	–18 to +5	–3.37
Talar first metatarsal (as seen in roentgenogram)	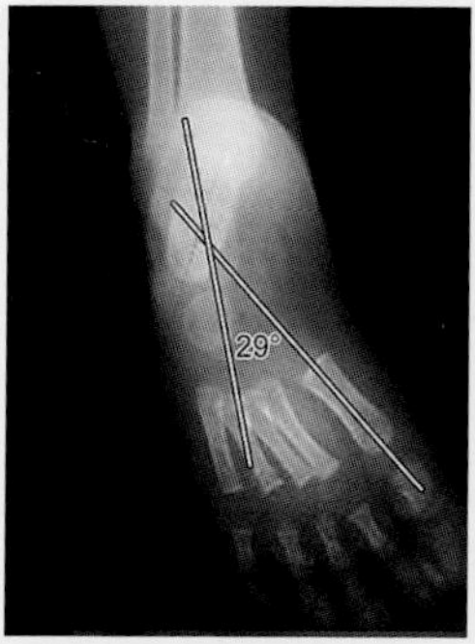 **Clubfoot**		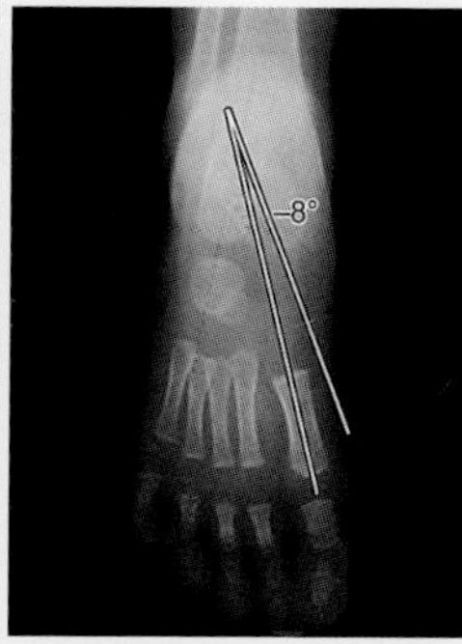 **Normal foot**	
Calcaneal fifth metatarsal (as seen in roentgenogram)	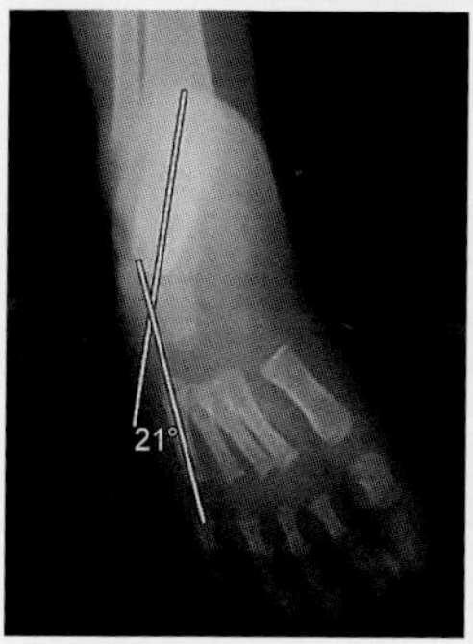 **Clubfoot**		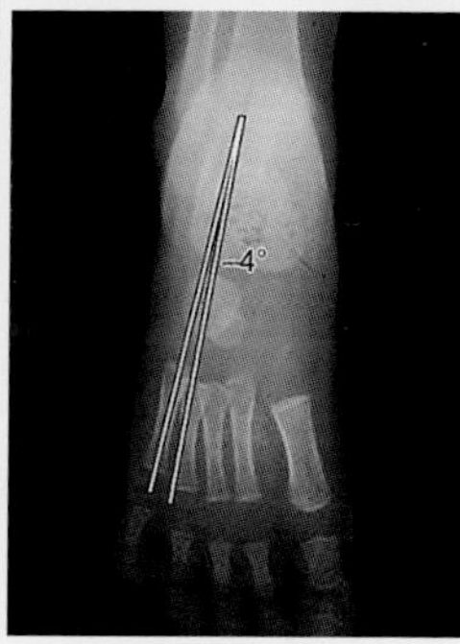 **Normal foot**	

FIG. 6.2B: Talar first metatarsal and calcaneal fifth metatarsal angle in clubfoot and normal foot with radiographs (Ponseti et al 1981)

Talar first metatarsal angle: A line through long axis of talus and another line through long axis of first metatarsal form the talar first metatarsal angle; a positive angle signifies adduction of the first metatarsal **(Fig. 6.2B)**.

Calcaneal fifth metatarsal angle: The calcaneal fifth metatarsal angle is formed by a line through long axis of calcaneus and another line through long axis of fifth metatarsal; a positive angle signifies adduction of fifth metatarsal **(Fig. 6.2B)**.

CHAPTER 7

Classification

CLASSIFICATION OF CLUBFOOT

Not all clubfeet are the same and it is important that all people treating clubfoot use the same terms to describe the different types. Each type of clubfoot has unique characteristics and may need specific treatment. Early recognition of the type of clubfoot one is dealing with can help to guide appropriate treatment. Although there is no universal classification system for clubfoot, clubfoot can be classified according to the nature of the deformity.

Positional Clubfoot

Positional clubfoot refers to a flexible foot that was held over time in an abnormal position in utero. When the child is born, due to the prolonged positioning, they may present with one or both feet in a resting position. Children with positional clubfoot typically exhibit unrestricted passive range of motion of forefoot and ankle. The foot at the time of birth has some deformity but bony alignment is not impacted, and foot position is likely corrected through conservative treatment involving a programme of stretching, range of motion, and weight bearing. In a small number of cases postconservative treatment, the foot

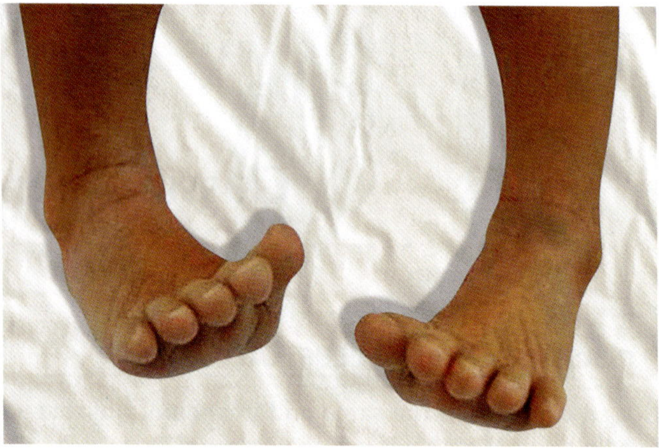

FIG. 7.1: Bilateral positional clubfeet

needs one or two casts to ensure that they are maintained in a corrected position although in the majority of cases these feet usually correct well and do not lead to any long lasting, significant impairment **(Fig. 7.1)**.

CLUBFOOT

It has been divided into idiopathic (isolated) and secondary (syndromic) clubfoot.

Idiopathic Clubfoot

Most commonly, clubfoot is classified as "idiopathic clubfoot" meaning there is no known cause for the deformity. In idiopathic clubfoot, there can also be a definite hereditary influence, in that if a person has a relative, parent, or sibling with clubfoot, then they are more likely to have clubfoot or have a child with it (3–10% chance). Within the group of idiopathic clubfeet there is a wide spectrum of impairment depending on severity, as well as whether the clubfoot has been untreated, partially treated, poorly treated, or successfully treated.

- *Untreated clubfoot:* All clubfeet from birth up to 2 years of age that have had very little or no treatment can be considered as untreated clubfeet **(Fig. 7.2A)**.
- *Treated clubfoot:* Untreated clubfeet that have been corrected with Ponseti treatment are termed "treated clubfeet". Treated clubfeet are usually braced full-time for 3 months and at night up to the age of 4 or 5 years **(Fig. 7.2B)**.
- *Recurrent/Relapsed clubfoot:* This is a clubfoot which has achieved a good result with Ponseti treatment, but the deformity has recurred. The most common reason is due to abandoning the braces early **(Fig. 7.2C)**.
- *Neglected clubfoot:* The neglected clubfoot is a clubfoot in a child older than 2 years, where little or no treatment has been performed. The neglected clubfoot may respond to Ponseti treatment, but also may have bony deformity that requires surgical correction **(Fig. 7.2D)**.

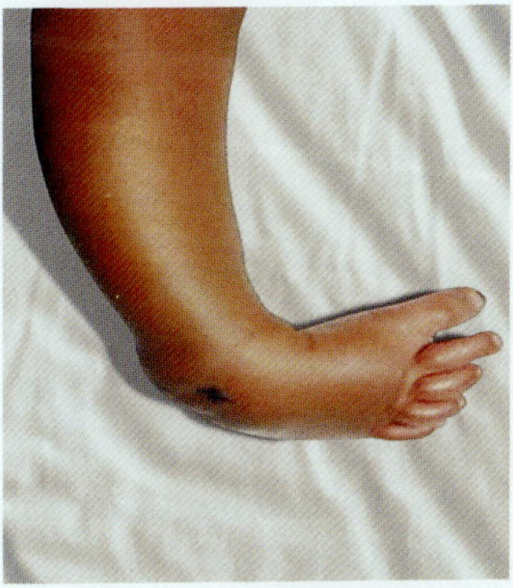

FIG. 7.2A: Untreated clubfoot

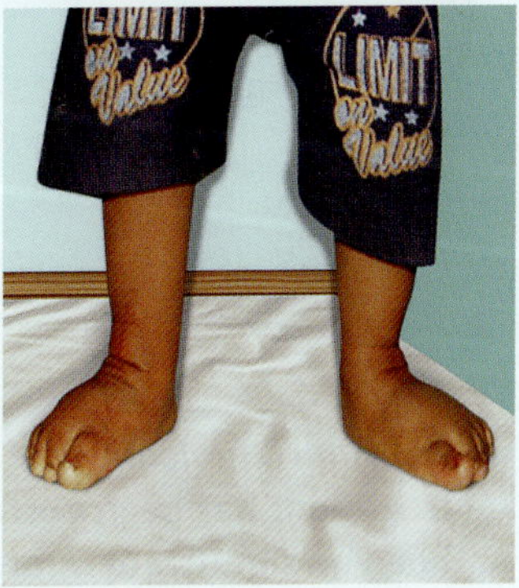

FIG. 7.2B: Treated clubfoot

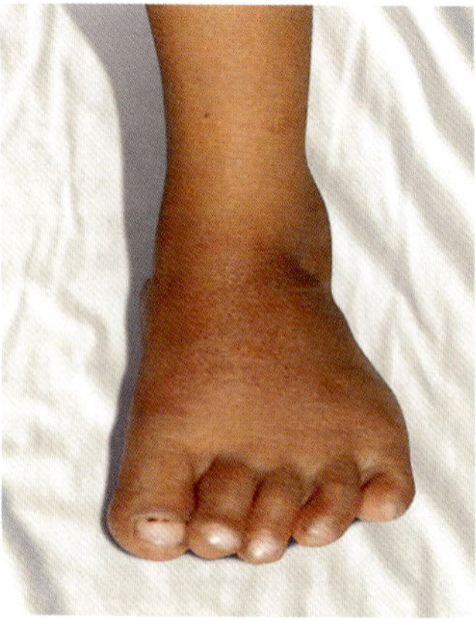

FIG. 7.2C: Relapse clubfoot

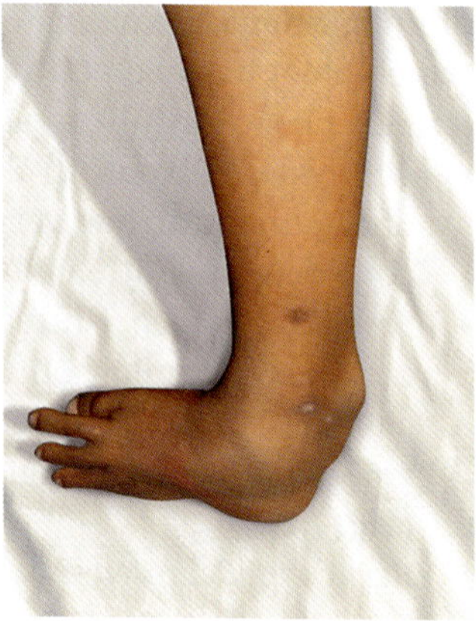

FIG. 7.2D: Neglected clubfoot

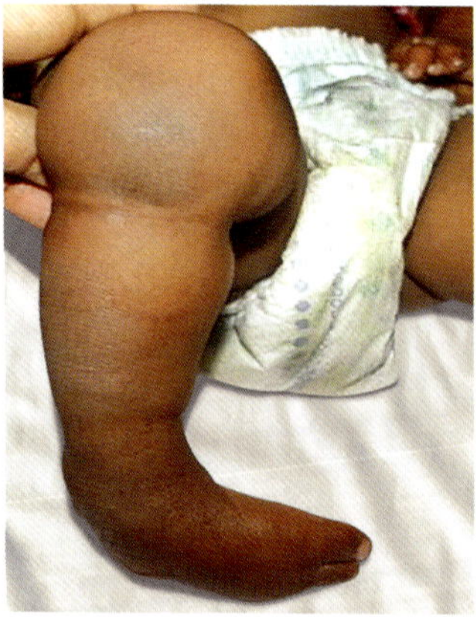

FIG. 7.2E: Resistant clubfoot

- *Resistant clubfoot:* This is a clubfoot where Ponseti treatment has been correctly performed but there has been no significant improvement **(Fig. 7.2E)**.

Secondary Clubfoot

In addition to idiopathic clubfoot, many other conditions and complex secondary clubfeet are present. On the other hand, it occurs when there is another disease or condition that is causing or linked to the development of clubfoot. Such conditions are usually "Neurogenic, Arhtrogryposis multiplex congenita, Tibial hemimelia, and Amniotic band syndrome."

Neurogenic Cause

Such as Spina Bifida associated with concurrent sensory and/or motor impairments.

Arthrogryposis Multiplex Congenita

This is a congenital condition where the child is born with a number of deformities of the joints.

Tibial Hemimelia

In tibia agenesis, there is failure of formation of a normal tibia. There is spectrum of presentations from complete absence to slightly short tibia.

Amniotic Band Syndrome

The cause of amniotic band syndrome is not fully clear, but children with this condition are born with tight skin and soft-tissue bands around their limbs, constricting blood and lymph flow and causing swelling.

Atypical Clubfoot

Atypical clubfoot is a complex variant of idiopathic clubfoot. Atypical clubfoot presents with some similar signs of idiopathic clubfoot but in greater severity. Atypical clubfoot is resistant to most standard management and modified approaches are regularly required (detailed discussion in atypical clubfoot chapter later).

DIMEGLIO CLASSIFICATION

Clubfoot deformity can be classified according to the age of the child, associated deformities, type and severity of the deformity, and treatment taken in the past (conservative or operative). The determination of initial severity index is an important factor for each component of talipes equinocavovarus. We favor the classification method of Dimeglio since it is more objective and reproducible method of scoring **(Figs. 7.3A to G)**.

Point Allocation to Each Deformity and Scoring of Clubfoot According to Dimeglio/Bensahel (1995)

Each major component of clubfoot (equinus, hindfoot varus, midfoot rotation, and forefoot adduction) is graded clinically from 4 to 1 (most severe to most mild). Additional points are added for posterior crease (PC), medial crease, cavus, and poor musculature. Total score is divided into four groups of severity, i.e., I, II, III, and IV (benign, moderate, severe, and very severe) **(Table 7.1)**.

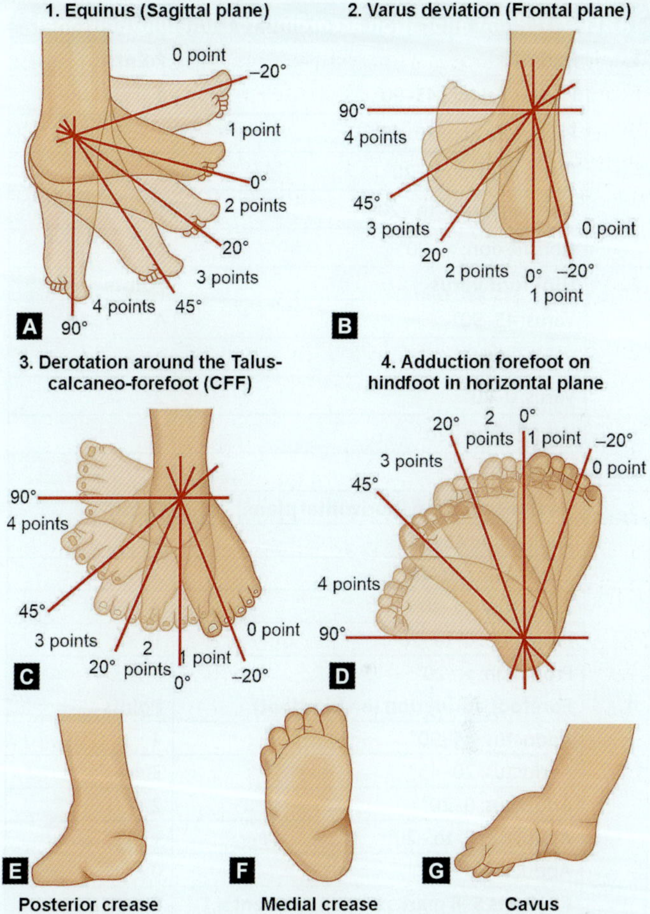

FIGS. 7.3A TO G: Pictorial representation of point allocation for the classification of clubfoot deformity according to Dimeglio/Bensahel

TABLE 7.1: Point allocation according to Dimeglio/Bensahel.

1.	**Equinus**	**Points**
	Plantar flexion: 45–90°	4
	Plantar flexion: 20–45°	3
	Plantar flexion: 0–20°	2
	Dorsiflexion: 0° to –20°	1
	Dorsiflexion: > –20°	0
2.	**Hindfoot varus**	**Points**
	Varus: 45–90°	4
	Varus: 20–45°	3
	Varus: 0–20°	2
	Valgus: 0° to –20°	1
	Valgus: > –20°	0
3.	**Midfoot rotation (horizontal plane)**	**Points**
	Supination: 45–90°	4
	Supination: 20–45°	3
	Supination: 0–20°	2
	Pronation: 0° to -20°	1
	Pronation: > –20°	0
4.	**Forefoot adduction (on hindfoot)**	**Points**
	Adductus: 45–90°	4
	Adductus: 20–45°	3
	Adductus: 0–20°	2
	Abductus: 0° to –20°	1
	Abductus: > –20°	0
	For Parts 5–8 mark points as present = 1 Absent = 0	**Points**

Continued

Continued

4.	Forefoot adduction (on hindfoot)	Points
	Adductus: 45–90°	4
	Adductus: 20–45°	3
	Adductus: 0–20°	2
	Abductus: 0° to –20°	1
	Abductus: > –20°	0
	For Parts 5–8 mark points as present = 1 Absent = 0	**Points**
5.	Posterior crease	0–1
6.	Medial crease	0–1
7.	Cavus	0–1
8.	Abnormal underlying musculature	0–1
	Total score	**Points**
	Type I (benign)	0–5
	Type II (moderate)	6–10
	Type III (severe)	11–15
	Type IV (very severe)	16–20

Equinus Deformity

If the foot is more or less fixed in any angle of plantar flexion from 0 position of the ankle it is "equinus deformity." In this condition the foot cannot be taken back even up to 0 position actively or passively.

According to classification of Dimeglio, the equinus deformity has been categorised from 0 to 4 points depending upon the angle of deformity **(Figs. 7.4A to F)**.

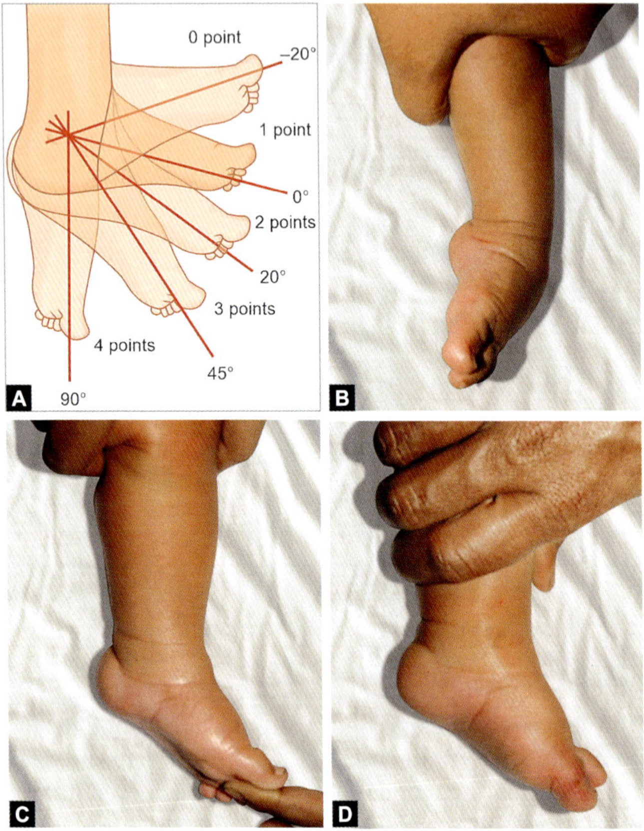

FIGS. 7.4A TO F: *Continued*

Continued

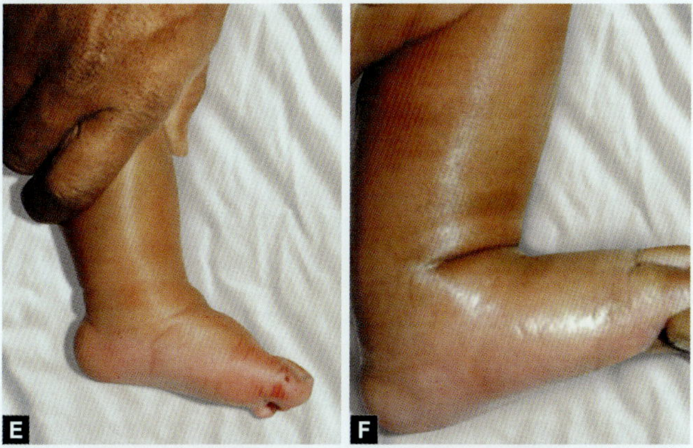

FIGS. 7.4A TO F: Schematic and photographic representation for point allocation to equinus deformity of clubfoot according to Dimeglio (1995)

Hindfoot Varus

Varus deformity of the heel is the result of contracture of ligaments, joint capsules, and tendons. It is seen in frontal plane when viewed from the back. The deformity is measured in 0–4 points **(Figs. 7.5A to F)**.

Midfoot Rotation (Horizontal Plane)

This is a horizontal plane evaluation of derotation of the calcaneopedal block. It is caused by soft-tissue contracture leading to abnormal position of the bone. The deformity is measured in 0–4 points **(Figs. 7.6A to F)**.

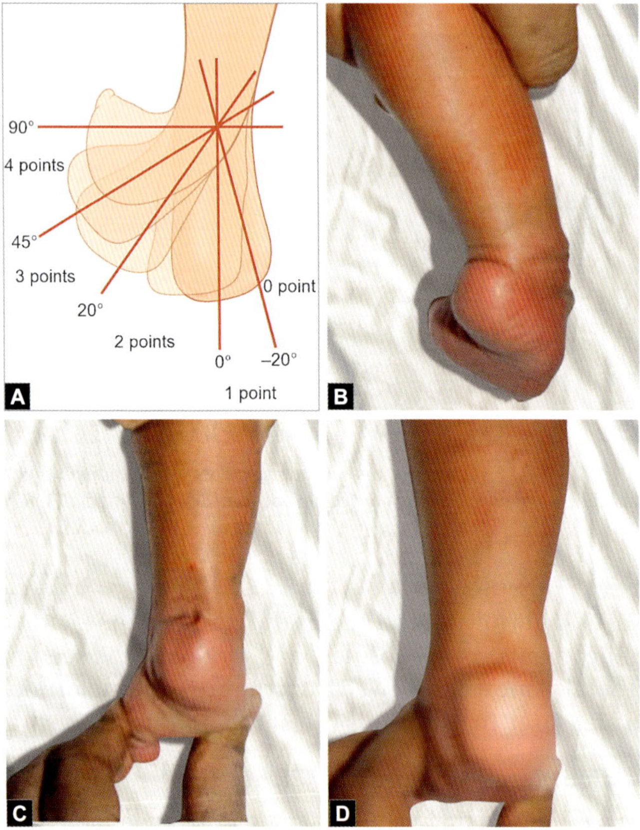

FIGS. 7.5A TO F: *Continued*

Continued

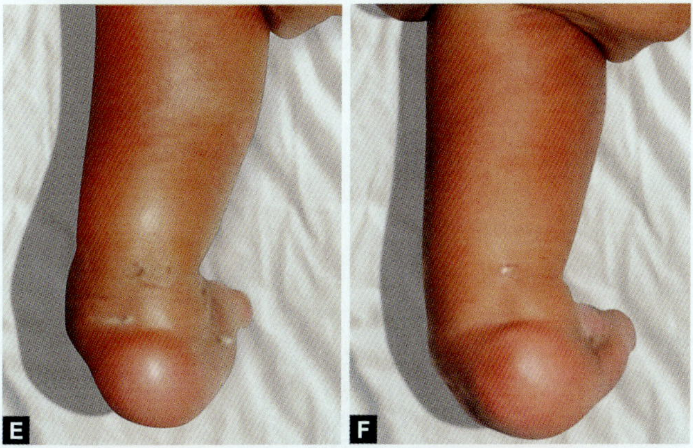

FIGS. 7.5A TO F: Schematic and photographic representation for point allocation to varus deformity of clubfoot according to Dimeglio (1995)

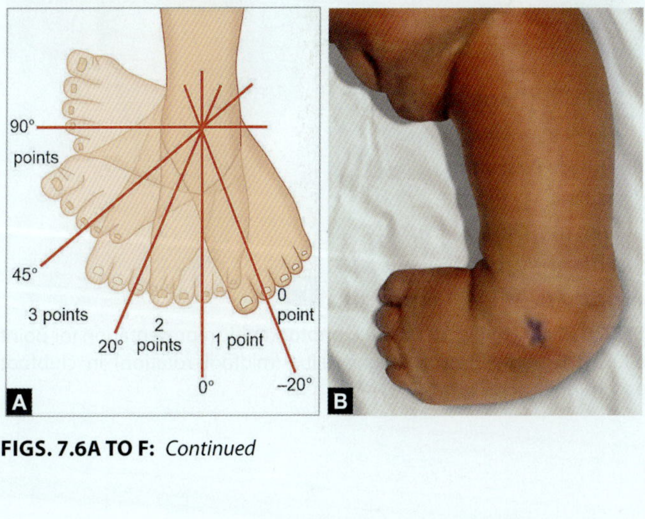

FIGS. 7.6A TO F: *Continued*

Continued

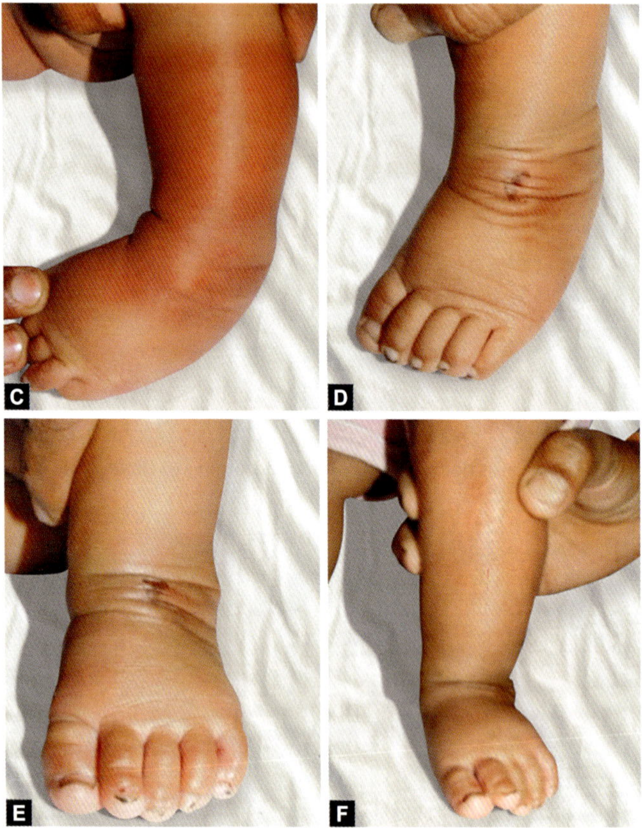

FIGS. 7.6A TO F: Schematic and photographic representation for point allocation to derotation around talus (midfoot rotation) in clubfoot according to Dimeglio (1995)

Forefoot Adduction (on Hindfoot)

The forefoot is adducted in comparison to the hindfoot. This is a horizontal plane deformity to be viewed from the plantar side of the foot **(Figs. 7.7A to F)**.

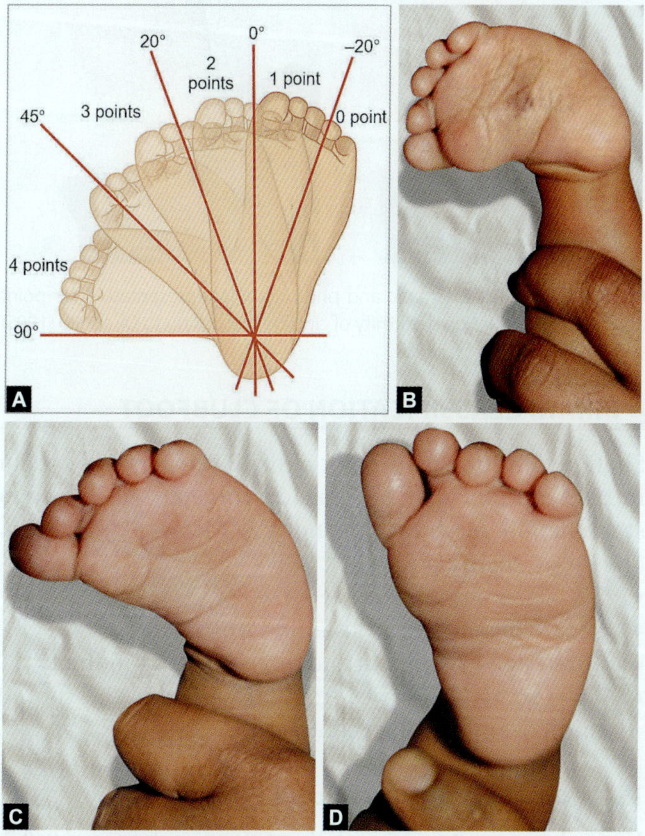

FIGS. 7.7A TO F: *Continued*

Continued

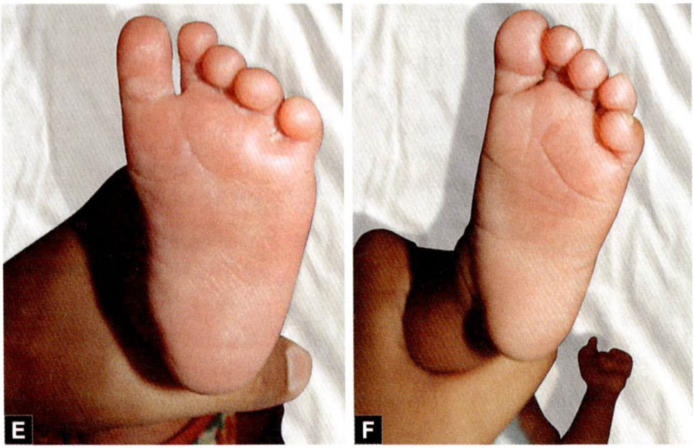

FIGS. 7.7A TO F: Schematic and photographic representation for point allocation to adduction deformity of clubfoot according to Dimeglio (1995)

PIRANI CLASSIFICATION OF CLUBFOOT

Shafique Pirani, the inventor of the Pirani scoring system in 1999, is a Canadian orthopaedic surgeon who helped to start clubfoot services in Uganda and Malawi.

The Pirani score key features:

- Six "signs" are assessed.
- Scored depending on severity—0, 0.5, or 1
- Three signs in midfoot and three signs in hindfoot
- Total score (TS) varies from 0 to 6 and is the sum of midfoot and hindfoot contracture scores.

Midfoot Contracture Score

Varies between 0 and 3 with three signs each scored 0, 0.5, or 1.

Medial Crease

- Gently correct the foot by lifting the foot holding the second toe.
- Assess the depth of the crease and the presence of other creases.
  Several fine creases: 0 **(Fig. 7.8A)**
  Two or three moderate creases: 0.5 **(Fig. 7.8B)**
  Single and deep crease: 1 **(Fig. 7.8C)**

Curved Lateral Border

- Make sure the child's foot is relaxed.
- Observe from the plantar aspect, and use a pen held against the lateral edge of the calcaneum.
- Assess the point on the lateral border of the foot at which it deviates from a straight line.
  Straight and without deviation: 0 **(Fig. 7.9A)**

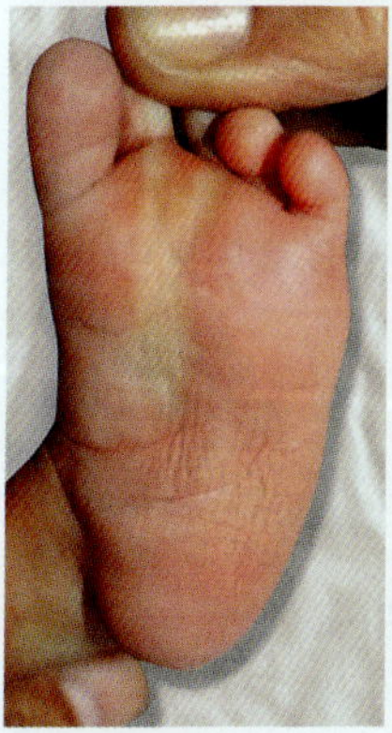

FIG. 7.8A: Multiple fine medial crease: 0

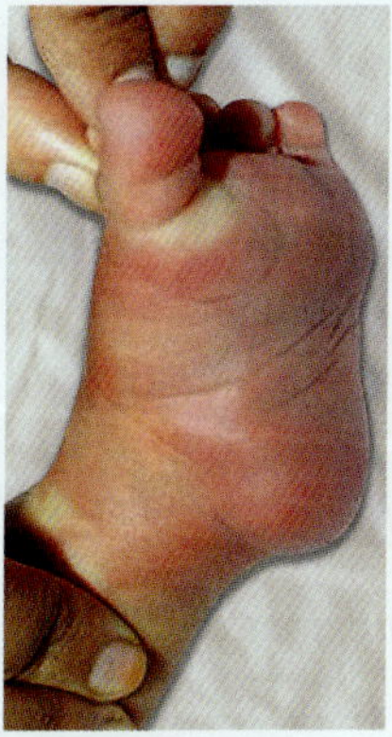

FIG. 7.8B: 2–3 Moderate medial crease: 0.5

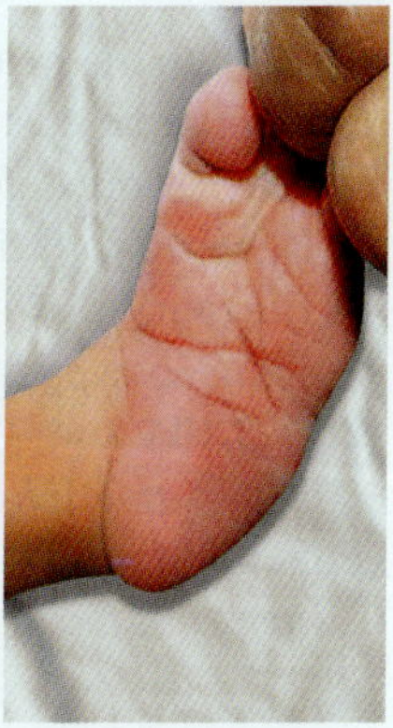

FIG. 7.8C: Single deep medial crease: 1

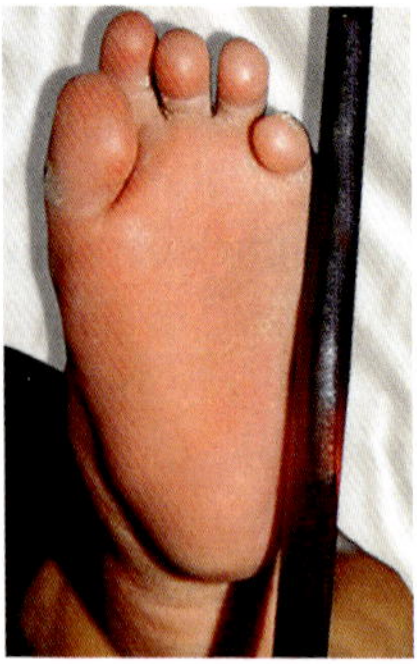

FIG. 7.9A: Straight lateral border: 0

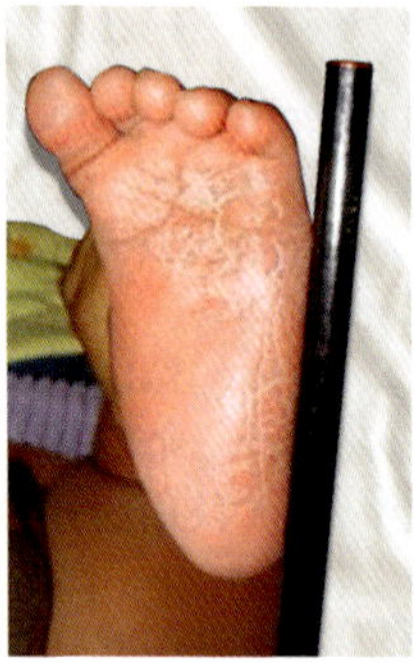

FIG. 7.9B: Deviates at metatarsals: 0.5

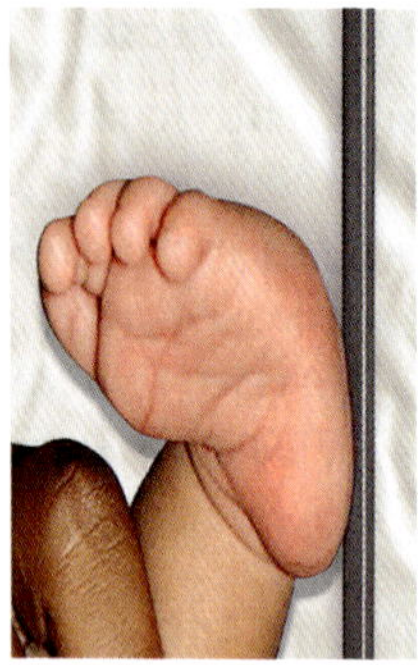

FIG. 7.9C: Deviates at calcaneo-cuboid joint lateral border: 1

Deviates at the level of the metatarsals: 0.5 **(Fig. 7.9B)**
Deviates at the calcaneo-cuboid joint: 1 **(Fig. 7.9C)**

Lateral Head of Talus

- Palpate the head of the talus with the foot uncorrected (it may be easier to find initially if you move the foot into a more deformed position).
- Keeping your finger/thumb on the talus, gently correct the foot.

Talus completely sinks under the navicular, score: 0 **(Figs. 7.10A and B)**

Moves partially but does not completely sink, score: 0.5 **(Figs. 7.10C and D)**

Remains fixed and does not sink: 1 **(Figs. 7.10E and F)**

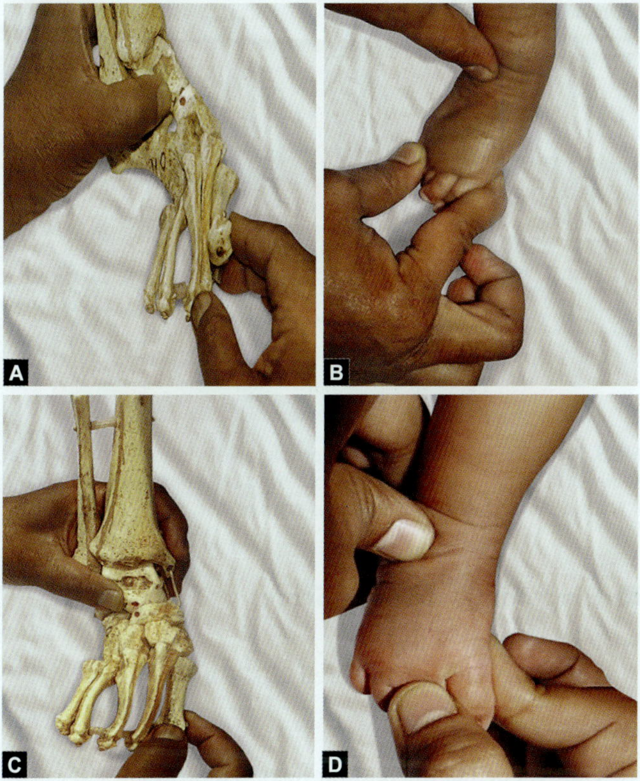

FIGS. 7.10A TO F: *Continued*

Continued

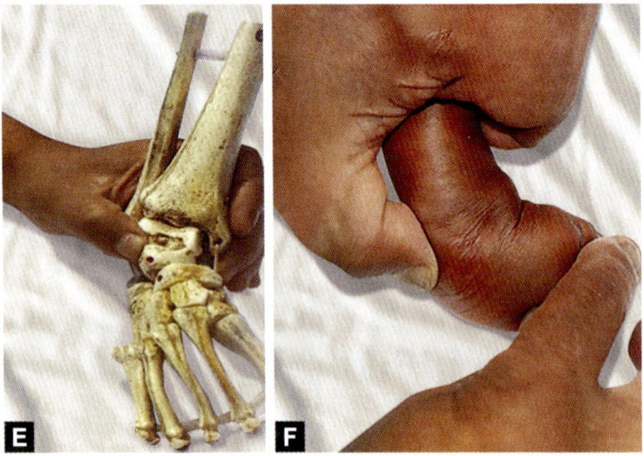

FIGS. 7.10A TO F: (A and B) Talus completely sinks under the navicular, score: 0; (C and D) Moves partially but does not completely sink, score: 0.5; (E and F) Remains fixed and does not sink: 1

Hindfoot Contracture Score

Varies between 0 and 3.

Three signs are each scored 0, 0.5, or 1.

Posterior Crease

- Gently correct the plantar flexion (equinus).
- Assess the depth of the crease and the presence of other creases.

  Presence of several fine creases: 0 **(Fig. 7.11A)**
  Two or three moderate creases: 0.5 **(Fig. 7.11B)**
  Single and deep crease: 1 **(Fig. 7.11C)**

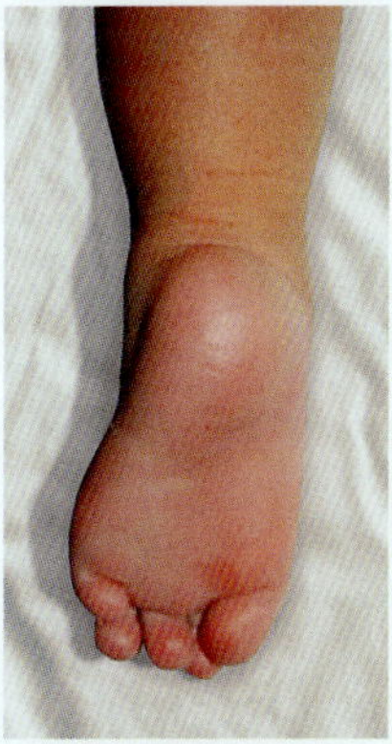

FIG. 7.11A: Multiple fine posterior crease: 0

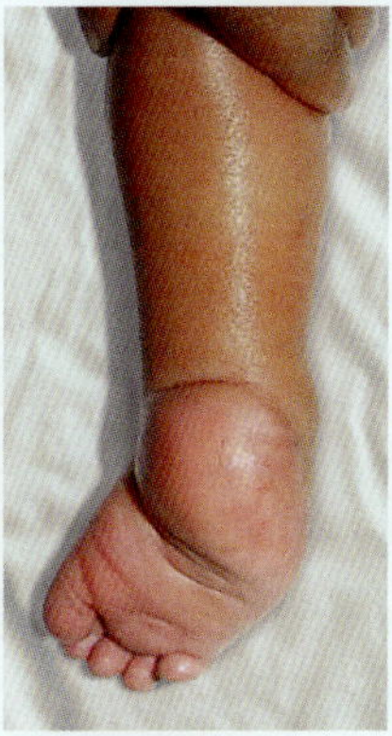

FIG. 7.11B: 2–3 moderate posterior crease: 0.5

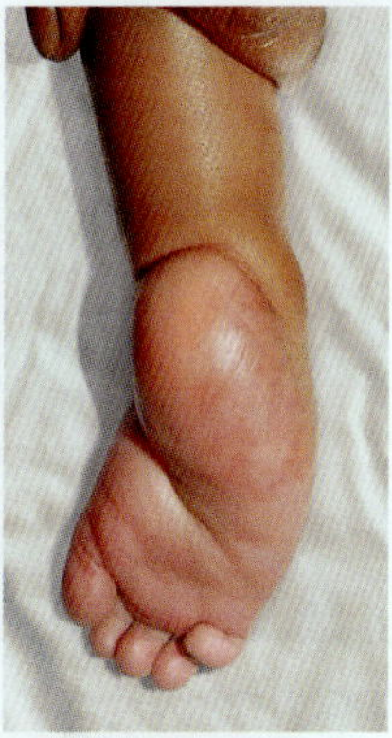

FIG. 7.11C: Single posterior deep crease: 1

Empty Heel

- Hold the foot in mild correction and palpate with a single index finger.
- Ascertain how much flesh there is in the heel between your finger and the calcaneum.

Easy to palpate the calcaneum, which is not far under the skin: 0 **(Fig. 7.12A)**

Calcaneum palpable which is just felt through a layer of flesh: 0.5 **(Fig. 7.12B)**

Deep under a layer of tissue, very difficult to feel: 1 **(Fig. 7.12C)**

(0 is like touching your own chin, 0.5 like touching the tip of your nose, and 1 like touching the soft part of your palm below the base of your thumb).

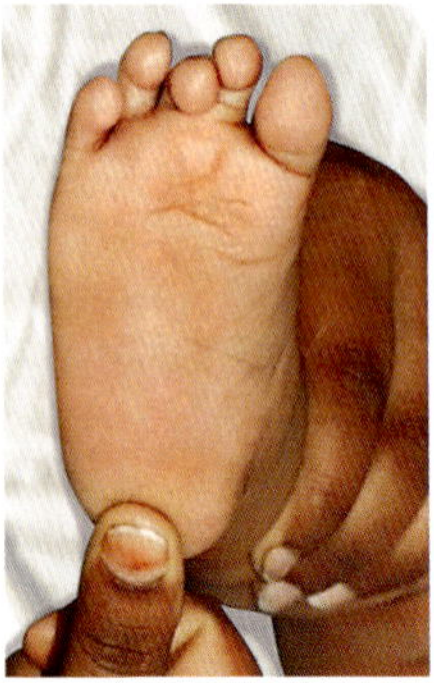

FIG. 7.12A: Empty heel: 0

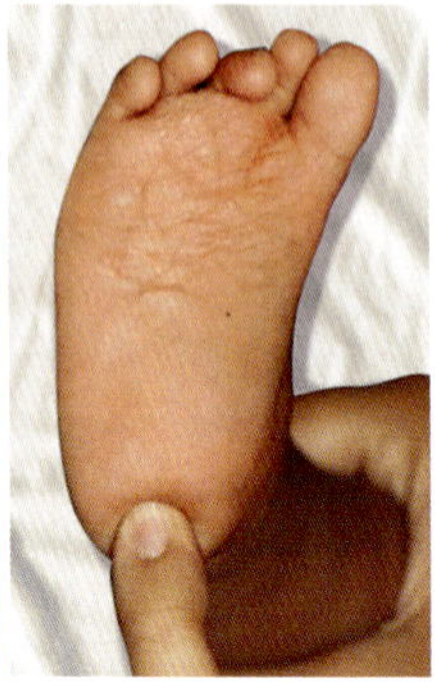

FIG. 7.12B: Empty heel: 0.5

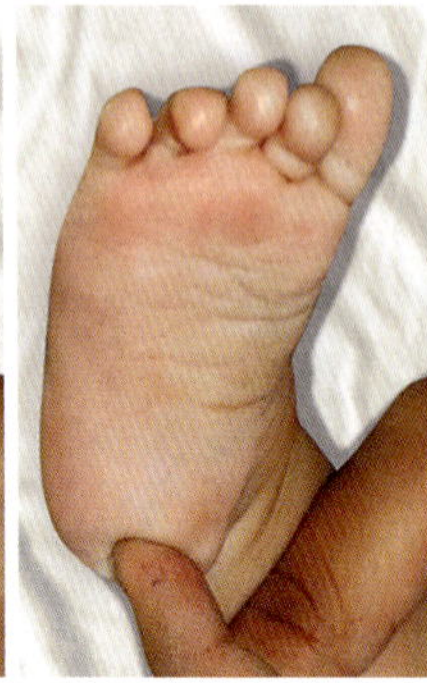

FIG. 7.12C: Empty heel: 1

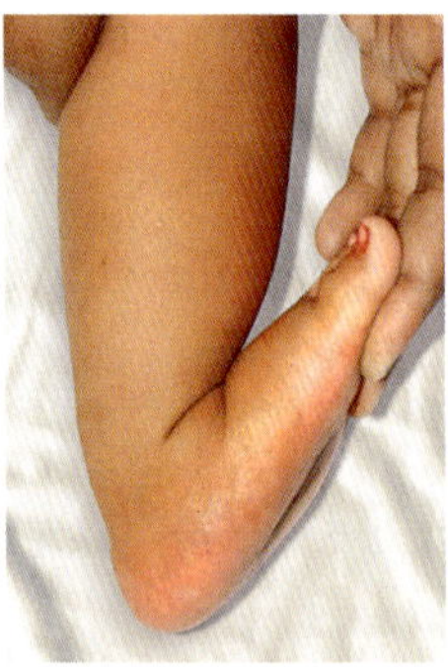

FIG. 7.13A: Dorsiflexion beyond plantigrade: 0

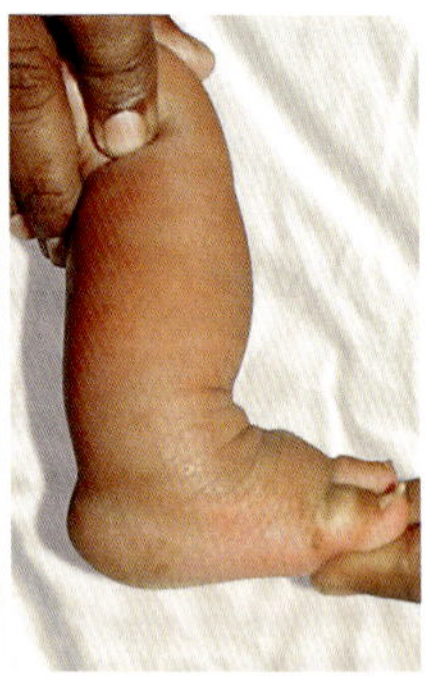

FIG. 7.13B: Able to reach plantigrade: 0.5

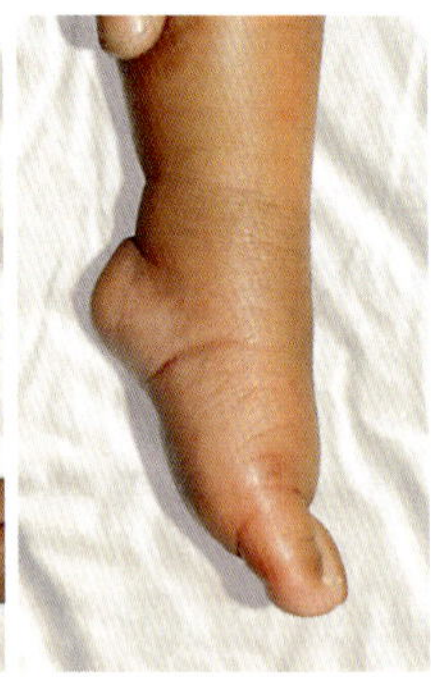

FIG. 7.13C: Foot in plantar flexion: 1

Rigid Equinus

- Correct the plantar flexion as much as is comfortable for the child, holding the knee straight.
- Assess the degree of dorsiflexion obtained.
  Able to dorsiflex beyond plantigrade: 0 **(Fig. 7.13A)**
  Able to reach plantigrade (or 90°): 0.5 **(Fig. 7.13B)**
  Unable to reach plantigrade (<90°): 1 **(Fig. 7.13C)**

PIRANI SCORE RECORD SHEET

The Pirani score should be recorded at each visit during the correction phase of clubfoot treatment. Most clinics have a paper form to record it. Below is an example of the Global Clubfoot Initiative Pirani Score Form. You will also find two other examples of Clubfoot Assessment Forms including the Global Clubfoot Initiative Pirani Score Form and the CURE Clubfoot Form to record and display the history, physical examination, and treatment in the Resource Section below.

It can indicate when foot is ready for tenotomy. The **Table 7.2** below shows the effects of Ponseti treatment and tenotomy on midfoot contracture score (MFCS), hindfoot contracture score (HFCS), and TS. The MFCS drops rapidly

TABLE 7.2: Pirani scores record sheet for a child at consecutive weeks.

Gender: Male			**Age: 12 days**	
Cast no.	1	2	3	4
Date/Month	5th	6th	8th	10th
Pirani score				
• Lateral border	1	0.5	0.5	0
• Medial crease	0.5	0.5	0.5	0
• Talar head	1	0.5	0	0
Midfoot score	2.5	1.5	1	0
• Posterior crease	0.5	0.5	0.5	0.5
• Empty heel	1	0.5	0.5	0.5
• Equinus	1	1	1	0.5
Hindfoot score	2.5	2	2	1.5
Total score	5	3.5	3	1.5

with manipulation and casting whereas HFCS remains high. The tenotomy is done in week 5 when the MFCS has dropped to "0", but HFCS remains >"1". After tenotomy, HFCS improves from 2.5 to 0.5, but does not correct completely.

CLINICAL SIGNIFICANCE

- It is helpful in assessing severity of deformity at the time of presentation and at each visit.
- It is helpful in assessing the response of clubfoot to pop cast treatment.
- Indirectly it helps in identifying underlying pathology (primary or secondary cause) based on response to pop treatment at each visit.
- Use of Pirani score to indicate tenotomy.

CHAPTER 8

Treatment

The goal of treatment is to correct all the components of the deformity in congenital clubfoot simultaneously except equinus and to achieve functional, pain free, normal looking plantigrade supple foot with good mobility which can fit into a normal shoe (without any modification). A totally normal foot is hard to achieve. Most of the orthopaedic surgeons believe that the initial treatment should be non-operative and must begin just after the birth to take advantage of favourable viscoelastic properties of the connective tissue forming the ligaments, joint capsules and tendons (Attlee-1868). Postero-medial soft tissue release and other surgeries are invariably followed by deep scaring with unhealthy and non-cosmetic look, especially in infants. The exact anatomical realignment is not possible even after capsular and ligamentous release. The talonavicular, talo-calcaneal and calcaneocuboid joint surfaces do not match even after surgery and any attempt to realign them makes joint surfaces incongruous. However, wire fixation through joint cartilage roughly aligns the position of bones and it causes further damage to articular cartilage.

PRINCIPLES OF PONSETI TECHNIQUE

Although all components of clubfoot except equinus are corrected simultaneously, it is essential to understand each deformity and their correction separately to inculcate this new concept of treatment.

Cavus

The cavus that is high medial arch is the first component to start with. In clubfoot, the first metatarsal shows excessive plantar flexion leading to pronation of forefoot in relation to hindfoot resulting in cavus deformity **(Fig. 8.1A)**. It is corrected by supinating the forefoot by lifting the head of first metatarsal with some abduction thereby placing the forefoot in proper alignment with the hindfoot **(Fig. 8.1B)**.

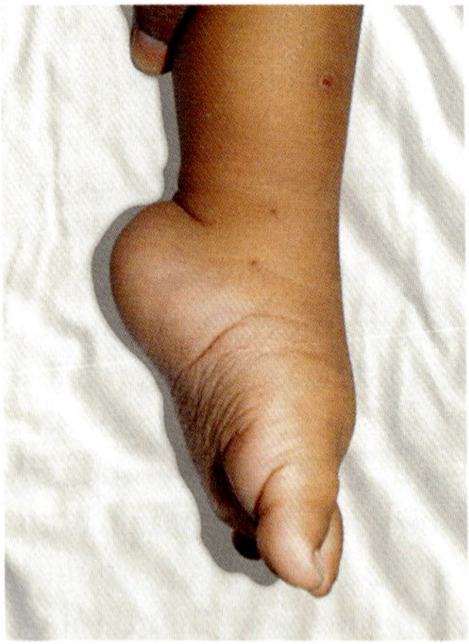

FIG. 8.1A: Untreated clubfoot showing cavus

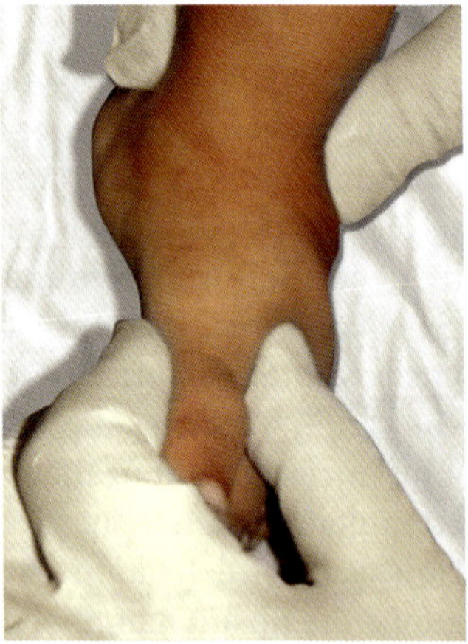

FIG. 8.1B: Supination by lifting the first metatarsal head to reduce cavus

As suggested by Dr Ponseti one must distinguish cavus from the rare plantaris deformity of foot in which all metatarsals are in about equal degree of plantar flexion with heel varus and adduction. This differentiation is essential for treating plantaris deformity since all metatarsals must be dorsiflexed simultaneously for correction in contrast with clubfoot where only first metatarsal is lifted.

Since plantar fascia and adductor muscles are stretchable and forefoot is flexible in infants, gentle manipulation of forefoot into supination and abduction usually corrects cavus deformity in the first cast.

In the first cast, forefoot is supinated by lifting the head of first metatarsal with some abduction which is done by keeping the thumb over the head of talus to bring it in proper alignment with the hindfoot. Sole of the foot should be molded to maintain normal height of the medial arch **(Fig. 8.1C)**.

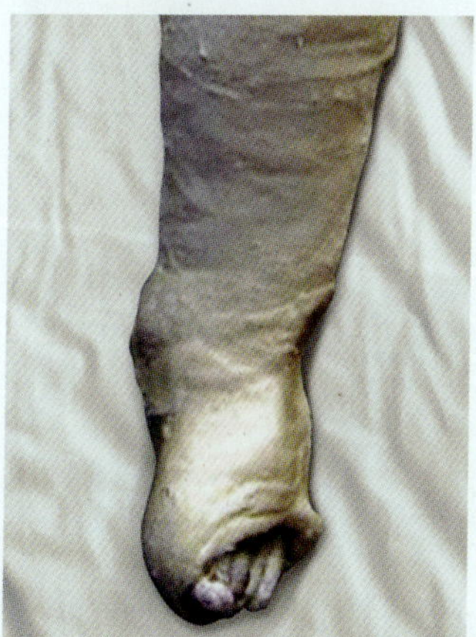

FIG. 8.1C: Molding of foot to maintain normal height of medial arch

Those cases, which do not respond to manipulation due to advanced age or some associated problems may need percutaneous plantar fasciotomy, followed by manipulations and serial casts to correct cavus.

Varus and Adduction

Foot is deformed in equinus, varus and adduction due to malpositioned talus, calcaneum, navicular and cuboid **(Figs. 8.2A and B)**. Owing to interdependence of tarsal joints, along with medial displacement of navicular, there occurs medial displacement and inversion of the cuboid and calcaneum; therefore, correction of adduction with fulcrum at the head of talus simultaneously corrects the varus of the heel.

The correction of cavus by supinating the forefoot brings metatarsals, cuneiforms, navicular and cuboid in

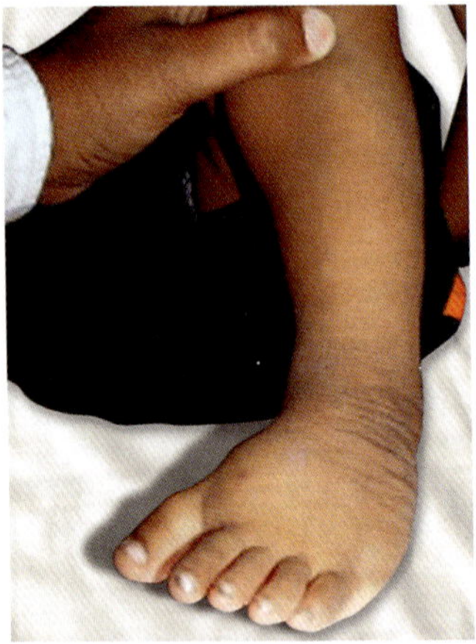

FIG. 8.2A: Untreated clubfoot showing adduction deformity

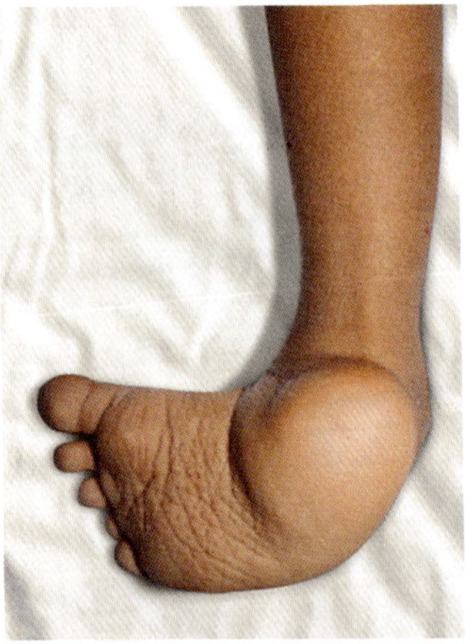

FIG. 8.2B: Untreated clubfoot showing heel varus

the same plane of supination. This converts whole of the foot into a lever arm with fulcrum at the head of talus. When pressure is applied over the head of talus and foot is abducted, the navicular abducts along with cuboid and calcaneus. Abduction of calcaneus leads to eversion of calcaneus as soon as it comes out from the undersurface of talus, correcting the heel varus. The motion starts at talonavicular joint, navicular pushing the cuboid, ultimately to calcaneum from internally rotated position to external rotation and from varus to neutral position. Thus, heel varus gets corrected along with forefoot adduction when the forefoot and midfoot are abducted. Heel is not touched during the entire manipulation. In most of the clubfoot cases, over-correction of heel varus is neither possible nor desirable.

Abduction is done by holding the forefoot in supination with counter-pressure applied on the lateral aspect of the head of talus with thumb **(Fig. 8.2C)**. After one to two minutes of gentle manipulation, a well-molded plaster cast upto upper third of thigh is applied.

Three to five plaster casts may be required to correct the adduction and varus. Care should be taken not to pronate the foot so as to prevent locking of calcaneum in varus under the talus. It is mandatory to achieve 60° to 70° of abduction before correction of equinus deformity by percutaneous tendo-Achilles tenotomy **(Fig. 8.2D)**.

In order to maintain strong abduction of the foot under the talus, the talus must be firmly immobilised against rotation in the ankle mortise and for this a high groin plaster cast is mandatory.

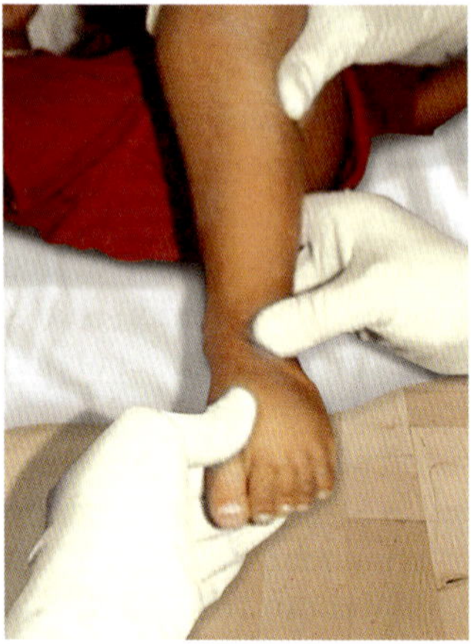

FIG. 8.2C: Manipulation: abduction is done by holding the forefoot in supination with counter pressure applied on lateral aspect of the head of talus with thumb

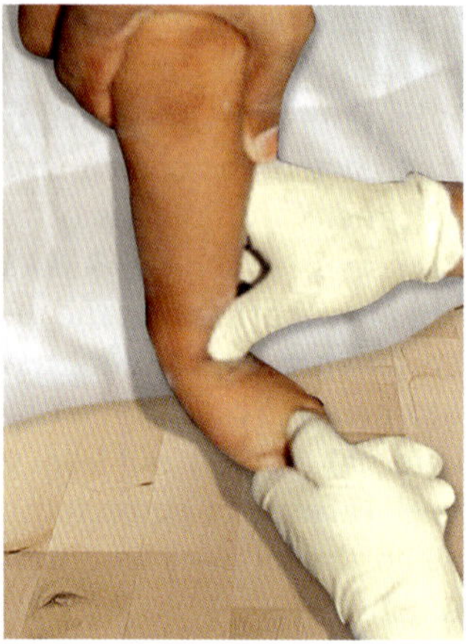

FIG. 8.2D: Manipulation: further abduction upto 70°

In severe clubfoot, complete reduction of the extremely medially displaced and inverted navicular may not be possible due to tight capsules, ligaments and deformed contour of talar head. Even with partially reduced navicular, the forefoot can be brought into proper alignment with hindfoot because naviculocuneiform and bifurcate ligaments yield and allow the lateral displacement and lateral angulation of the cuneiforms with respect to the navicular.

In spite of all care, relapses are common in severe clubfoot cases with partially reduced navicular. If relapse occurs, transfer of tibialis anterior tendon to the third cuneiform should be considered.

Equinus

Equinus deformity denotes position of foot in plantar flexion from zero position of ankle where foot cannot be taken back to zero position actively or passively. The hindfoot always remains off the ground. Further in most of the cases of the equinus deformity the culprit is tight tendo-Achilles and tight plantaris accentuated by the tightness of posterior capsule of the ankle and subtalar joint **(Fig. 8.3A)**.

Equinus is the last deformity to be corrected after correcting varus and adduction **(Fig. 8.3A)**. Equinus is corrected by stretching tight posterior capsule, ligaments and tendo-Achilles tendon. Foot is dorsiflexed with one hand under the entire sole and heel is grasped with the thumb and index finger of the other hand to pull it downward **(Fig. 8.3B)**. The heel can also be pulled downward with the bent index finger over tendo-Achilles insertion **(Fig. 8.3C)**.

After manipulations, if the tendo-Achilles is stretchable, two to three plaster casts are required to correct equinus deformity. During cast application the heel should be molded properly; while dorsiflexing the foot pressure should be applied on entire sole of foot to avoid rocker-bottom deformity. After achieving 15° or more dorsiflexion, last plaster is given with foot in 60° to 70° of abduction and cast is kept for 3 weeks.

In most of the cases, tendo-Achilles is very tight and stretching is not possible in first manipulation. In these cases percutaneous tendo-Achilles tenotomy should be performed under local anaesthesia as an outdoor procedure and final plaster cast is given in 15° to 20° dorsiflexion

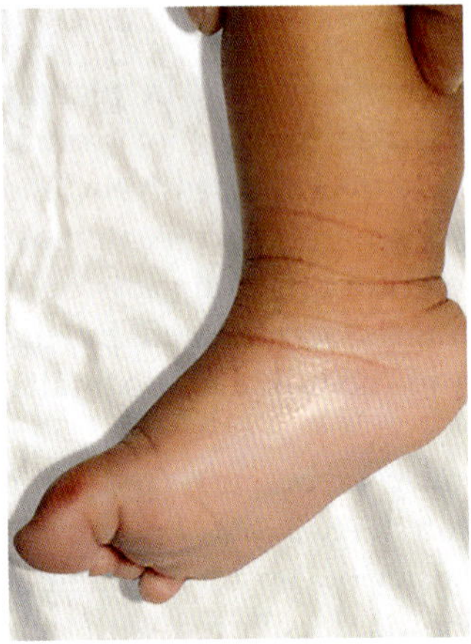

FIG. 8.3A: Clubfoot showing equinus deformity

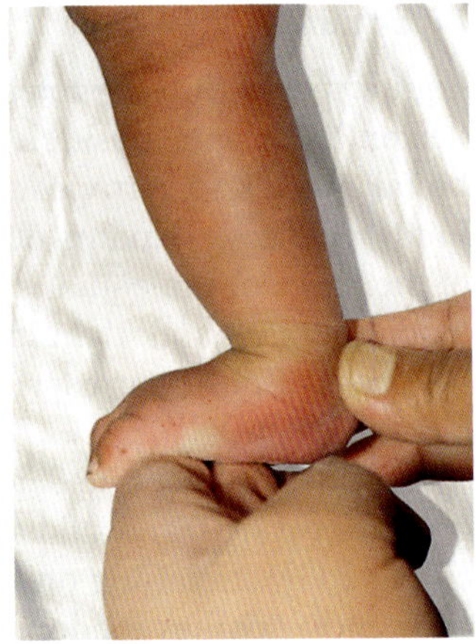

FIG. 8.3B: Heel pulling with thumb and index finger

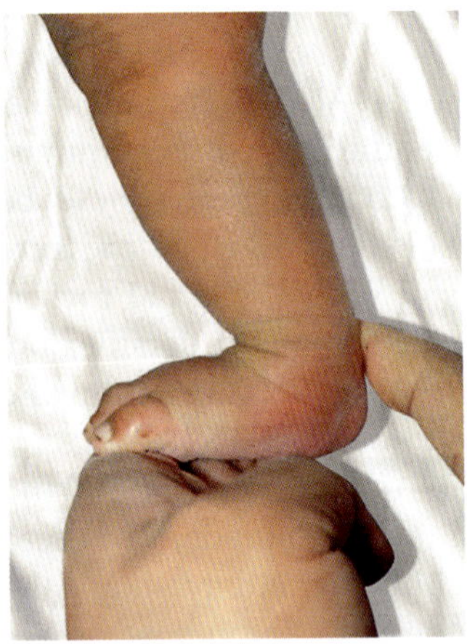

FIG. 8.3C: Heel pulling with curved index finger

with 60° to 70° abduction for 3 weeks. Thereafter, the foot is kept in about 70° of external rotation with the help of shoes attached to a bar for several months in order to prevent retraction of medial tarsal ligaments.

Tibial Torsion

Hutchins et al (1986) observed that lateral malleolus is displaced backward in spite of medial tibial torsion. Krishna et al (1991) studied ultrasound scans of proximal and distal posterior tibial planes in normal children and in children with clubfeet.

They measured angular differences between proximal and distal posterior tibial planes. In their study normal children have a mean external tibial torsion of 40° whereas children with clubfoot have a mean external tibial torsion of only 18°.

Thus, children with clubfoot have no internal torsion rather they have only half of the external tibial torsion as compared to normal children.

With advancement in imaging techniques, now tibial torsion can be measured more accurately with the help of computerised tomography **(Figs. 8.4A to C)**.

Posterior displacement of lateral malleolus can also be the result of wrong manipulation of foot into abduction with the heel in inversion and adduction under the talus. It is also produced when the child walks with uncorrected heel varus and adduction, where he turns his foot laterally to avoid tripping causing further displacement of lateral malleolus. It can be avoided by correcting the adduction and varus by keeping the thumb over the head of talus in supinated foot during abduction.

Tibial torsion, heel varus and foot adduction can be gradually corrected by the above knee cast with knee in 90° of flexion. Splints with shoes in external rotation for many months maintain the correction of internal tibial torsion.

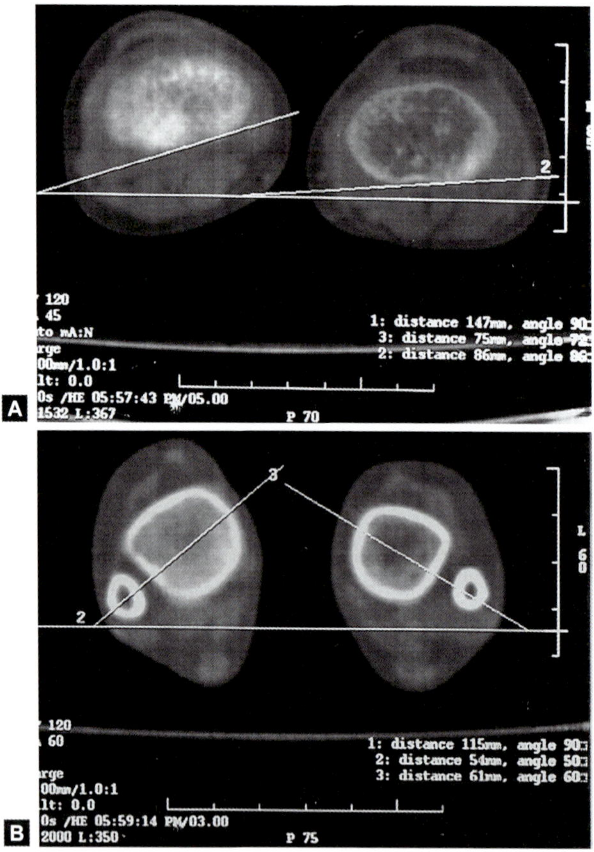

FIGS. 8.4A TO C: *Continued*

Continued

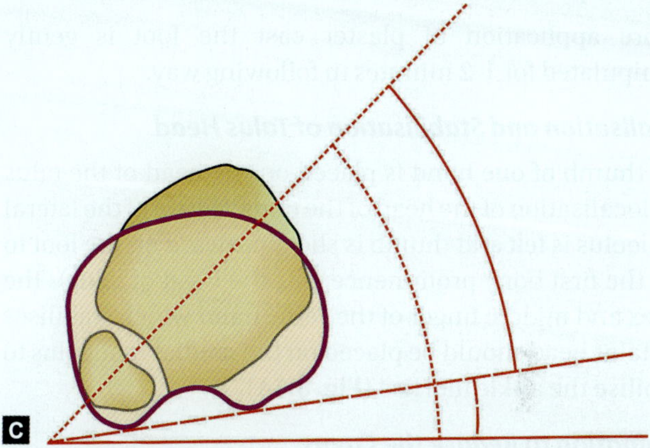

FIGS. 8.4A TO C: (A) Axial CT image of the proximal tibia just above the head of fibula. The tangent to the dorsal border forms the proximal line of reference, (B) Axial scan of distal tibia just above the ankle joint. The distal line of reference is formed by the pilon centre point, i.e., the midpoint of the circle that fits into the tibial pilon includes the fibular notch of the tibia but excludes the medial malleolus, and the mid point of a line over the fibular notch, (C) Proximal line of reference (......) and distal line of reference (—) form an angle with the horizontal line. Subtraction of the proximal from the distal angle results in the angle of tibial torsion (solid arc)

STEPS OF PONSETI TECHNIQUE

Treatment should start immediately after birth. Most of the clubfoot can be corrected by manipulation and serial cast application which should be continued till full correction is achieved. Approximately five to six casts are required to correct adduction and varus at an interval of one week. After correcting these deformities equinus deformity is corrected by percutaneous tendo-Achilles tenotomy and final cast is applied for 3 weeks.

Manipulation

Before application of plaster cast the foot is gently manipulated for 1–2 minutes in following way:

Localisation and Stabilisation of Talus Head

The thumb of one hand is placed on the head of the talus (for localisation of the head of the talus, the tip of the lateral malleolus is felt and thumb is slided forward on the foot to feel the first bony prominence, i.e., the head of talus). The index and middle finger of the same hand which stabilises the talar head should be placed on the medial malleolus to stabilise the ankle mortise **(Fig. 8.5A)**.

Supination to Reduce the Cavus

The cavus, which means high medial arch, requires only supination of forefoot to achieve normal longitudinal arch of the foot. There are two methods of manipulation:

1. *Two hand method*: Thumb of one hand is placed over the head of talus and forefoot is held with thumb of other hand on dorsal and index finger on plantar aspect of head of first metatarsal. Supination is done by lifting the head of first metatarsal as shown in **Figures 8.5B and C**.
2. *One hand method*: In this method thumb is placed on the plantar and medial surface of head of 1st metatarsal and index finger of the same hand is placed on the lateral aspect of head of talus and the forefoot is supinated with the help of thumb, as shown in **Figure 8.5D**. The other hand can be used to mold the cast as required.

Correction of Adduction

To correct adduction, abduction of foot is performed gradually up to 60° to 70° with thumb over the head of talus and holding forefoot with thumb and index finger of other

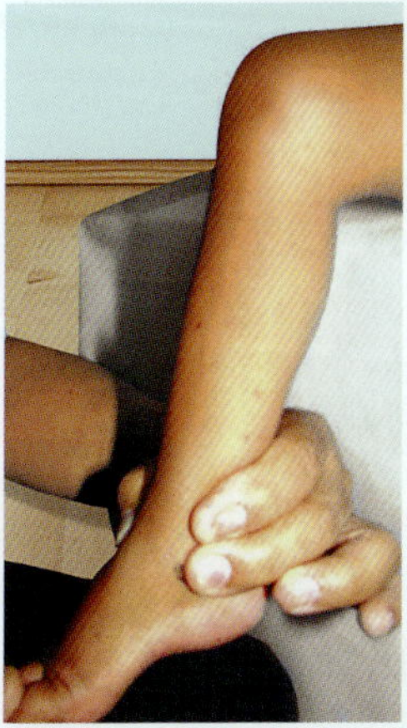

FIG. 8.5A: Method of stabilisation of talar head

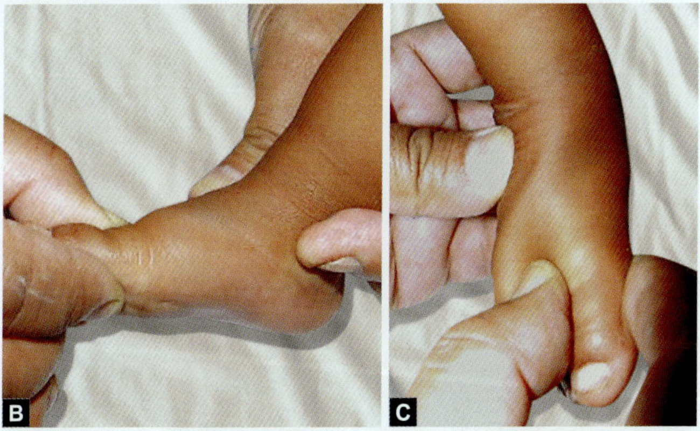

FIGS. 8.5B AND C: Supination of forefoot (medial view and frontal view) two hand method

hand gently without causing discomfort to the child. Care should be taken to keep the forefoot in supination, as soon as the foot is abducted, supination decreases but the foot is never pronated in the whole manoeuvre **(Figs. 8.5E and F)**.

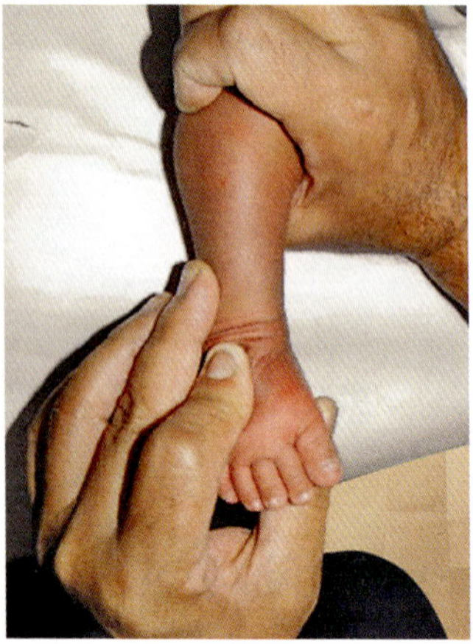

FIG. 8.5D: Supination of forefoot (one hand method)

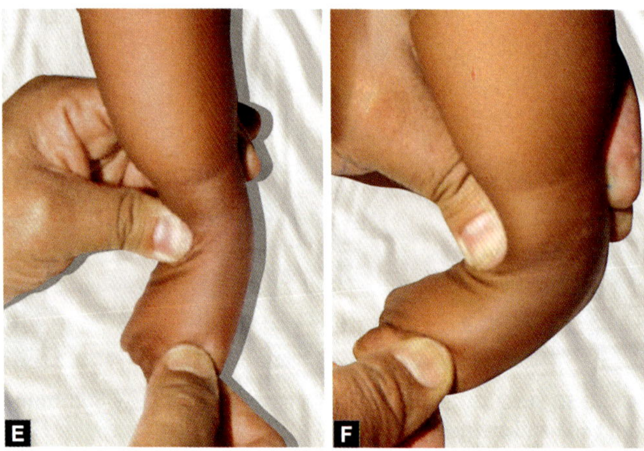

FIGS. 8.5E AND F: Correction of adduction: outward pressure is exerted on the metatarsals and counter pressure on the lateral aspect of the head of talus; The foot is gradually abducted to 70°, supination is decreased but foot is never pronated

Assessment of Adequate Abduction

Before performing tendo-Achilles tenotomy, we must confirm that foot is sufficiently abducted.

There are three methods to assess the desired abduction:

1. Ability to palpate anterior process of calcaneum (the best sign): In the clubfoot the calcaneum is rotated internally beneath the talus and anterior process of calcaneum is not palpable. As the foot is abducted the calcaneum is rotated externally and anterior process of calcaneum is palpable.
2. Abduction of approximately 60° to 70° in relation to the frontal plane of tibia
3. Neutral or slight valgus of calcaneum

Correction of Equinus

If correction of equinus is not possible by heel pulling and manipulation then percutaneous tendo-Achilles tenotomy is needed to correct equinus deformity as shown in **Figures 8.7A to H**.

Plaster Cast Application

The mother and the surgeon should make the baby comfortable. The baby should be kept on one end of the table to provide space for the mother and the assistant on the other side. The baby should be fed before manipulation. Mother should be allowed to remain close to the baby during all manipulations and plaster application.

The foot is manipulated first approximately for 1–2 minutes before application of plaster cast. During plaster application, the assistant holds the thigh with one hand and toes with thumb and index finger of the other hand, maintaining the knee in 90° of flexion **(Fig. 8.6A)**. A two-inch wide cotton soft roll is applied starting at toes and proceeding upward to the upper thigh. Care should be taken that the cotton roll should cover half of the width to get double thickness over the skin and especially over the heel. Extra cotton should be avoided rather proper molding should be done to avoid loosening of plaster cast. The cotton should be applied snugly over the foot and ankle and loosely over the calf and thigh to avoid extra pressure **(Fig. 8.6B)**.

A two inch or four inch wide plaster bandage depending upon the age of the child is wrapped snugly over the foot and ankle for better molding and loosely over calf and thigh to avoid excessive pressure on muscles **(Fig. 8.6C)**. The plaster is started from toes and is extended below the knee. While the assistant holds the foot, the orthopaedic surgeon should apply the plaster himself from toes extending up to the knee.

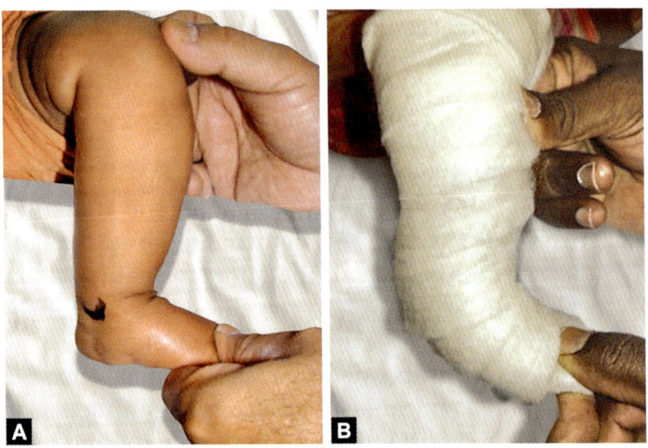

FIGS. 8.6A AND B: Assistant holds the foot and cotton roll being applied

The toes are covered by the assistant's thumb and finger so that the plaster bandage covers the thumb to prevent crowding of toes. Now, the surgeon takes over the foot from the assistant for correction and proper molding especially over the arch of the foot and heel **(Figs. 8.6D and E)**.

The molding is done gently with anatomical precision; the cast covering the toes should be flattened to maintain the neutral position. The heel prominence should be molded precisely **(Fig. 8.6D)**. The thumb should not be kept on wet cast for a longer time to avoid pressure sores. At the same time, the ankle and melleoli are well molded and the correction is done gently to avoid strain over the ligaments and joints. The heel should never rest on surgeon's hand or any tough structure otherwise it will lead to flattening of plaster over the heel. The heel should always be put in neutral position so that it does not go in valgus position. The molding is done at the sole of the foot to maintain normal height of medial arch **(Fig. 8.6E)**.

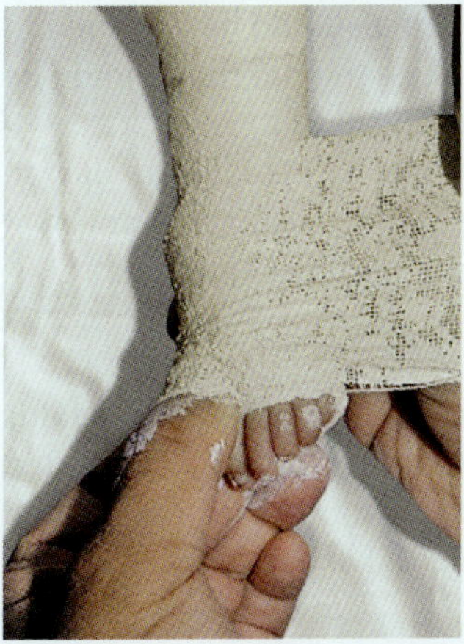

FIG. 8.6C: Application of plaster bandage by the surgeon with assistant sitting on medial side, holding the toes with one hand and thigh with other hand

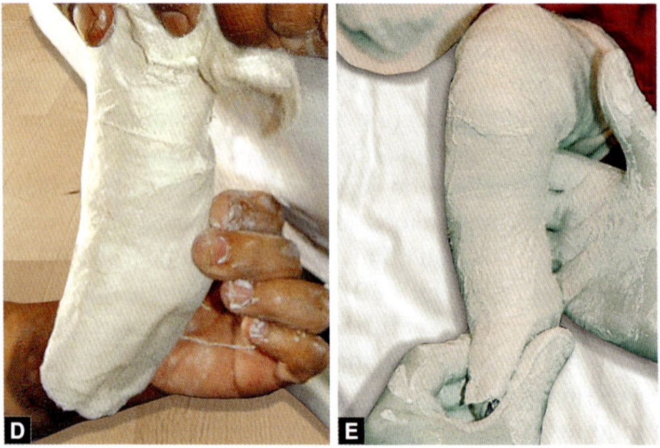

FIGS. 8.6D AND E: (D) Proper molding of heel prominence, (E) molding of medial arch of foot to maintain anatomical position

After molding and setting of below knee cast, plaster cast is extended above knee just below the groin with the knee at 90° flexion. Plaster cast should be trimmed in such a way that toes are free to expand but they should be prevented from plantar flexion **(Fig. 8.6F)**.

Change of cast can be done at every fifth day in newborns. After the age of one month, casts are changed at one week's interval till full correction is achieved.

First Cast

The first cast is applied with the thumb on the head of talus and forefoot is supinated by elevating the head of the first metatarsal by putting the thumb on dorsal aspect and index finger on plantar and medial aspect of head of first metatarsal **(Fig. 8.6G)**.

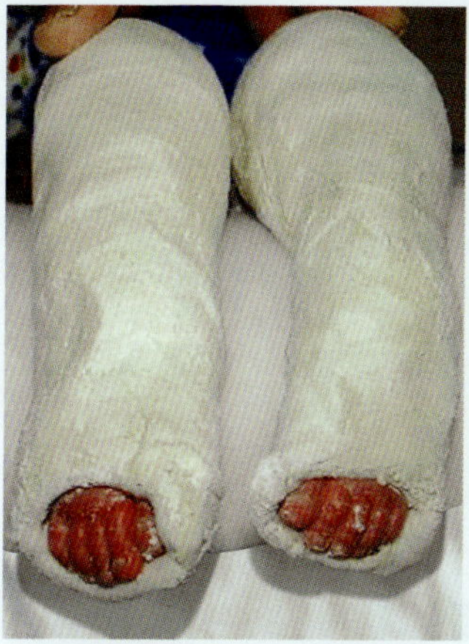

FIG. 8.6F: Trimming around toes to allow them to expand with plantar support to prevent toe flexion

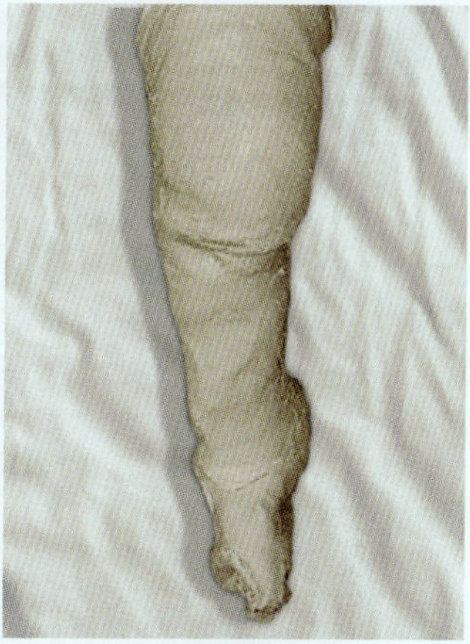

FIG. 8.6G: First cast is given with forefoot in supination

Second to Fifth Cast

During this phase of treatment the adduction and varus are fully corrected and navicular covers the anterior surface of the head of talus, which can be assessed by measuring the distance between medial malleolus and navicular tuberosity that is around 1.5 to 2 cm. During this phase abduction of foot is done by putting thumb of one hand on the head of talus and the thumb of other hand on dorsal aspect and index finger on plantar and medial aspect of head of first metatarsal and abduction up to 70° is achieved gradually. All casts are above knee and applied in two steps, firstly, below the knee then extending up to thigh. The foot is never pronated **(Figs. 8.6H to K)**. Heel should not be touched during the entire manipulation.

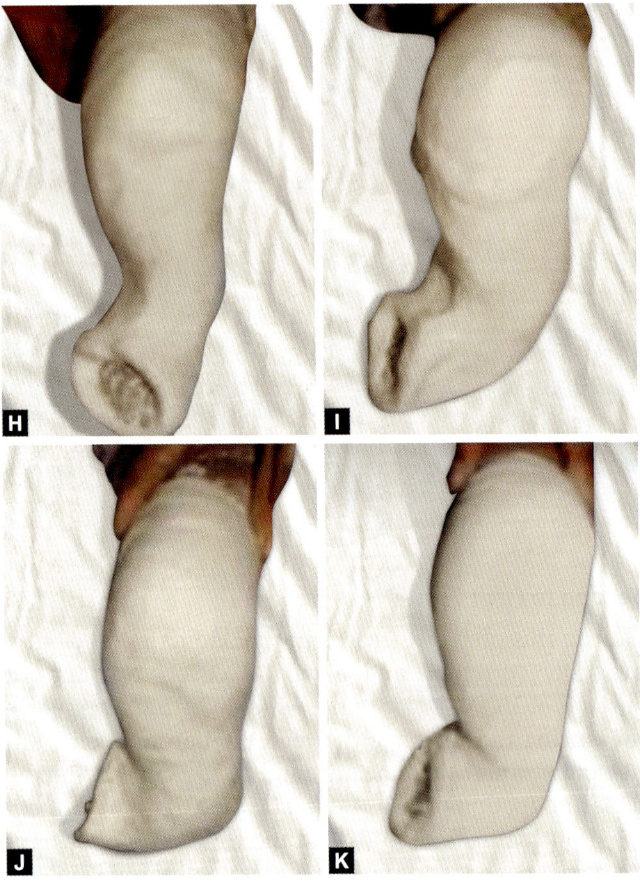

FIGS. 8.6H TO K: Second to fifth cast showing gradual abduction up to 70° without pronating the forefoot

Final Cast

Equinus is corrected after correction of adduction and varus deformities **(Fig. 8.6L)**. It is done by stretching the tight posterior capsule, ligaments and tendo-Achilles tendon. Foot is dorsiflexed with one hand under the entire sole and heel is grasped with the thumb and index finger of the other hand to pull it downward **(Fig. 8.6M)**. The heel can also be pulled downward with the bent index finger over tendo-Achilles insertion **(Fig. 8.6N)**.

After manipulations, if the tendo-Achilles is stretchable, two to three plaster casts are required to correct equinus deformity. During cast application the heel should be molded properly. While dorsiflexing the foot, pressure should be applied on entire sole of foot to avoid rocker-bottom deformity. After achieving 15° or more dorsiflexion,

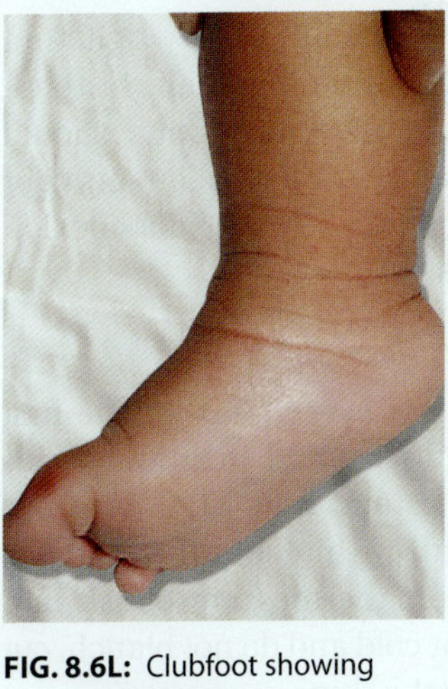

FIG. 8.6L: Clubfoot showing equinus deformity

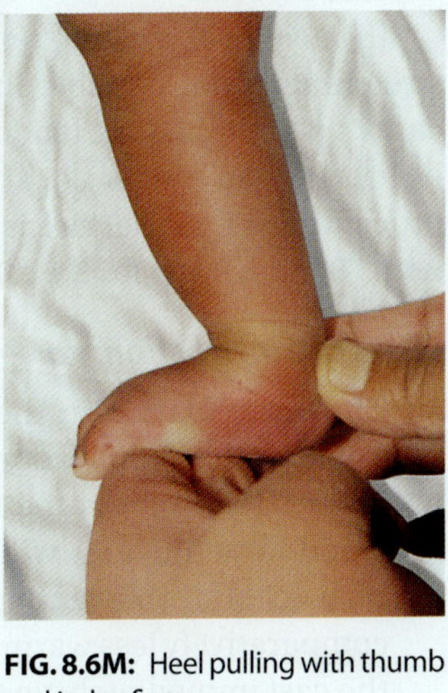

FIG. 8.6M: Heel pulling with thumb and index finger

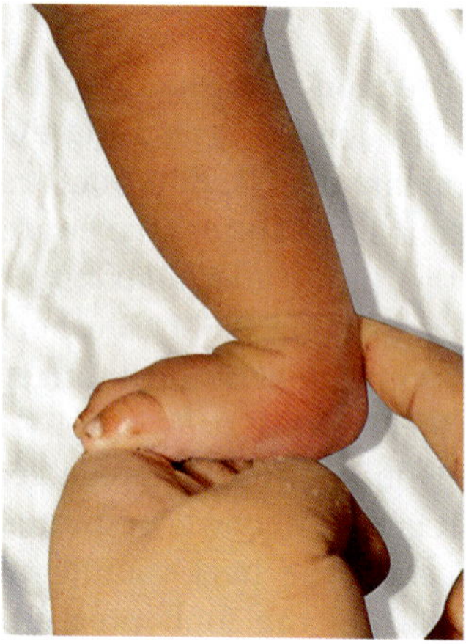

FIG. 8.6N: Heel pulling with curved index finger

last plaster is given with foot in 70° of abduction and cast is kept for 3 weeks.

In most of the cases, tendo-Achilles is very tight and stretching is not possible in first manipulation. In these cases percutaneous tendo-Achilles tenotomy should be performed under local anaesthesia as an outdoor procedure and plaster cast is given in 15° to 20° dorsiflexion with 70° abduction for 3 weeks.

Cast Care Instructions for Parents

1. Check circulation in the foot every hour for the first 6 hours after application of cast and then four times a day. Gently press the toes and watch the return of blood flow. The toes will turn white and then quickly turn to pink (blanching). If the toes are bluish and comparatively less warm or cold and do not blanch, cut the cast immediately up to the skin.

2. Note the relationship between the tips of the toes and the end of the cast. If the toes shrink back inside the cast, which means that the cast has slipped down and correct pressure on the foot is not being maintained. This might create pressure-sores and therefore change the cast.
3. Keep the cast dry and clean.
4. The cast should be placed on a soft pillow or on a rolled towel until it is dry and hard.
5. Use disposable diapers and change the diapers often to prevent soiling of the cast.

Tendo-Achilles Tenotomy

It is an outdoor procedure. Skin preparation of leg and foot is done from all aspects. One mL of 2% xylocaine is infiltrated around the tendon. The tendon is palpated about 1–2 cm above its insertion and tenotomy is performed with no.15 B.P. blade. A 'pop' is felt as the tendon is cut. An additional 10° to 15° of dorsiflexion is achieved immediately after tenotomy.

The post tenotomy cast is applied with foot abducted 60° to 70° in respect to the frontal plane of the tibia and 15° to 20° dorsiflexion. This cast is left in place for 3 weeks **(Figs. 8.7A to H)**.

BRACING AND PHYSIOTHERAPY

To get a functionally and cosmetically good foot, the treatment should not be limited only to manipulation and immobilisation. The accepted method to prevent relapse and rigidity in foot is proper use of brace and regular physiotherapy in the form of exercise and massage.

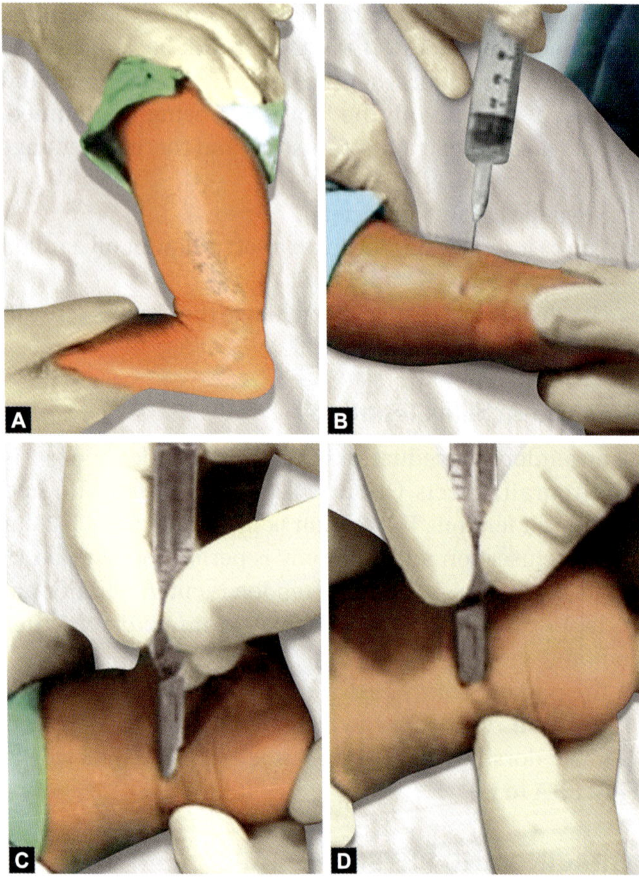

FIGS. 8.7A TO D: (A) Positioning of the foot before tenotomy, (B) Infiltration of local anaesthetic agent (Xylocaine 2%), (C) Stab incision, (D) Rotation of scalpel blade to 90° to perform tendo-Achilles tenotomy

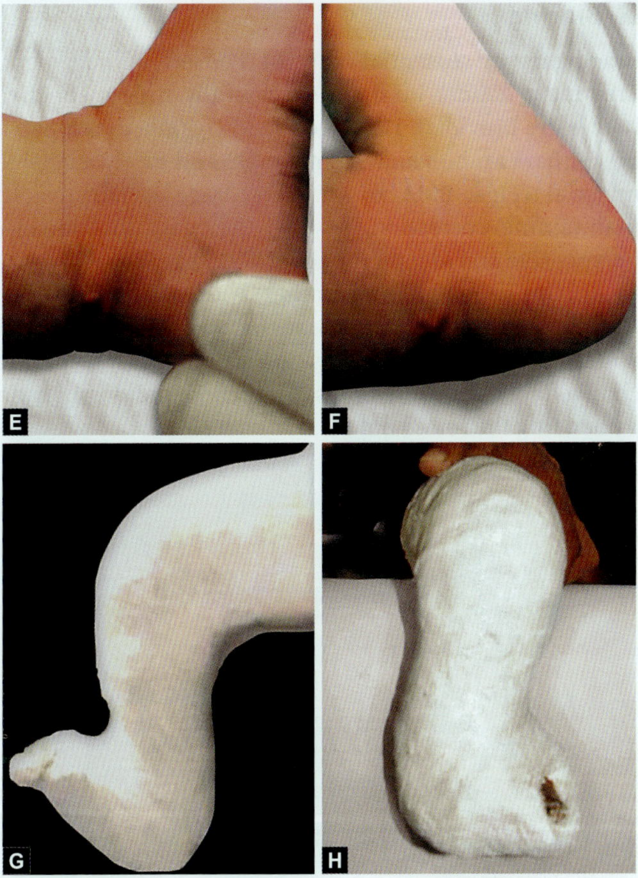

FIGS. 8.7E TO H: (E) Post tenotomy appearance of stab incision, (F) Correction of equinus, (G-H) Postoperative cast with full dorsiflexion (20°) at ankle and 70° abduction

Bracing

Bracing is an essential part of Ponseti management. Treatment cannot be done successfully unless effective braces are provided. HM Steenbeck, Uganda developed a brace that can be made from simple and easily available material **(Figs. 8.8A to C)**. This brace is effective in maintaining correction, easy to use, easy to fabricate, inexpensive and ideally suited for widespread use.

This brace has open-toe leather shoes with lace closures. A round metal bar holds the shoes in 70° of external rotation and 10–15° of dorsiflexion. Position of both the shoes can be changed towards more or less abduction and dorsiflexion by bending the round bar close to shoes.

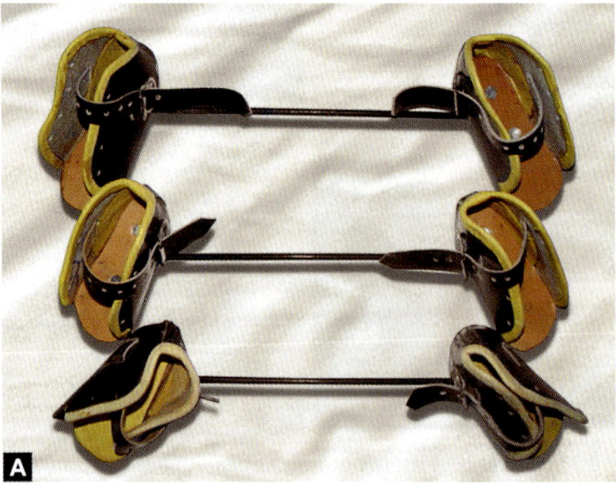

FIGS. 8.8A TO C: *Continued*

Continued

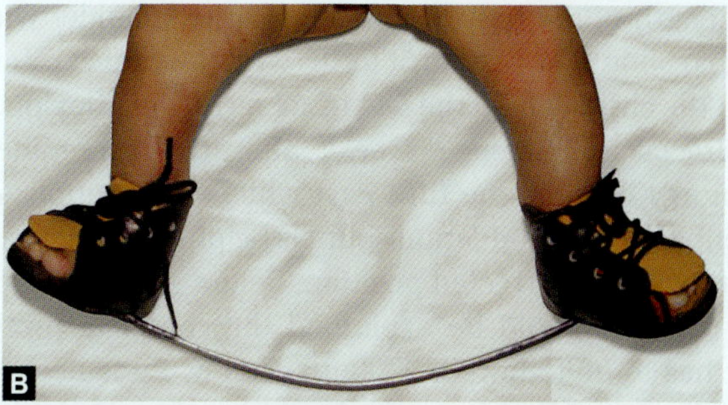

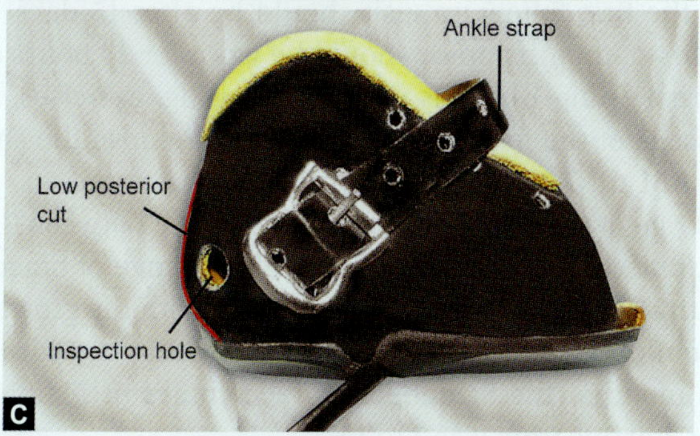

FIGS. 8.8A TO C: Photographs showing Steenbeck braces of different sizes, Bracing after full correction with Ponseti technique, Details of the shoe

The shoes have an inspection hole on the medial side of a well-molded heel counter to confirm that the heel adjusts itself properly into the shoes. The heel counter has a low posterior cut (in contrast to high top shoes), which prevents the heel from slipping out from the brace **(Fig. 8.8C)**. Brace is applied immediately after the removal of last cast.

For unilateral case—70° of external rotation on the clubfoot side and 45° of external rotation on the normal side

For bilateral case—70° of external rotation on both sides

Length of the bar should be equal to shoulder width. The bar should be bent to 5° to 10° with the convexity away from the child to hold the feet in 10° to 15° dorsiflexion.

Braces are given 3 weeks after the percutaneous tenotomy or after the fifth cast whichever is applicable. Steenbeck's foot abduction splint is helpful in maintaining the foot in the corrected position. Before giving the brace, the parents should be explained the complete protocol that has to be followed. A regular follow-up is necessary and the first follow-up visit should be after 15 days. For the first 3 months brace should be worn for 23 hours and the remaining 1-hour is used for cleaning, exercises, and massage of the foot. Our protocol is to remove the shoes at 7 AM till 7.30 AM to perform cleaning, exercises, and massage of the foot, again repeat the same between 7 PM to 7.30 PM **(Figs. 8.8D to H)**. Regular change of braces is required as the size of the foot changes with the growth of the child. Usually braces are replaced within the duration of 3 months. The Steenbeck's brace comes in 7 different sizes starting from size 7 to 13.

After 3 months the brace is used for 12 hours during night time only when the child is asleep, this provision is made to allow the toddler to walk during day hours or when he is awoken. To maintain correction, high top walking shoes are given along with night brace for 2–4 years. It is unnecessary to give any special shoe as it is ineffective in either case whether the foot has been corrected or not. Following full correction of the clubfoot, long-term monitoring is done. Child should be followed every 3 months for 2 years, thereafter; yearly follow-up is advised for 8–10 years to check any possible long-term relapse.

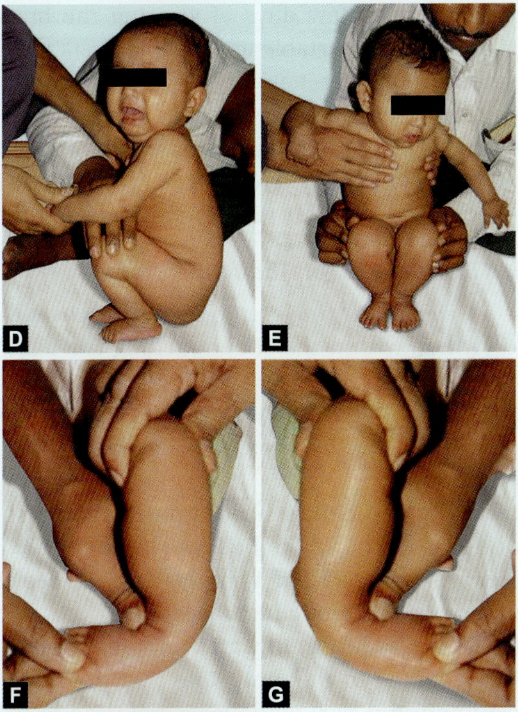

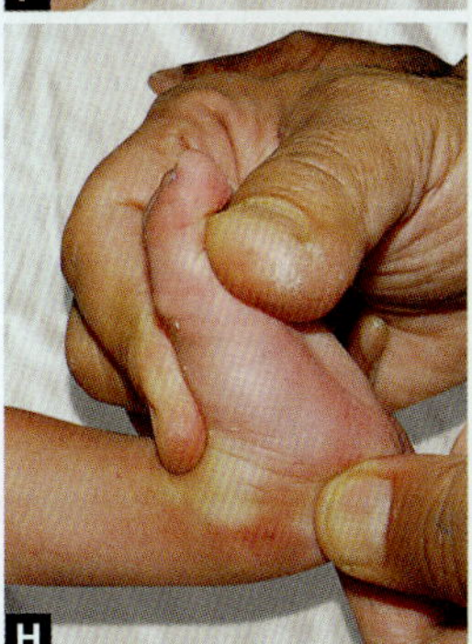

FIGS. 8.8D TO H: (D and E) Squatting with knees together and heel touching the ground for 5 minutes; (F and G) Place your thumb over anterior and lateral aspect of the ankle and with other hand hold the great toe and then gently move the foot in outward direction as shown in the photograph; (H) Move the foot upward slowly with full contact with sole and heel

During the first few days of wearing the brace, the baby may be uncomfortable as he/she adjusts to the legs being tethered together. It is very important that the brace should not be removed. After few days, the baby will adapt to the splint. Foot abduction brace is used only after the clubfoot has been completely corrected by manipulation, serial casting and, possibly tendo-Achilles release.

Wearing Instructions for Abduction Brace

1. Use always well-fitting cotton socks that cover the foot everywhere within the shoe touching the baby's foot and leg.
2. Hold the foot into the shoe and tighten the ankle strap first. This strap helps to keep the heel firmly down into the shoe.
3. Check that the child's heel is down in the shoe by pulling up and down on the lower leg. If the toes move backward and forward it indicates that heel is not down, so we must retighten the strap.
4. Lace the shoes just tightly, to keep the shoes well and firmly adapted to the foot. Note that the strap is the most important part while laces are used to hold the foot into the shoes.

Make sure that all the baby's toes are straight and none of them is bent. It is better to cut the distal portion of socks to visualise all the toes.

Physiotherapy

The mother should be taught to administer the exercises. The main exercises include stretching of tendo-Achilles tendon and connective tissues of the medial aspect of the foot. It has been observed that early intervention yields good results **(Figs. 8.8D to H)**.

EVALUATION IN SERIAL PLASTER CASTS

Clinical Evaluation in Serial Plaster Casts

Usually 5–6 casts are sufficient for correction of the deformities but sometimes more casts are needed in older children. The results of the manipulation and plaster casts depend on many factors:

1. Age of the child
2. Type of the foot with mild, moderate, severe and very severe deformity.
3. Time of starting the treatment, an early treatment gives better results.
4. Manipulation for one or two minutes before plaster casts is a must; if manipulation is not done, it becomes difficult to correct the deformities during plaster phase because the child cries a lot.
5. Plaster should be done with gentle manipulation. If abnormal pressure is applied during plaster application, it gives abnormal strain to the ligaments, even sometimes greenstick fracture of the metatarsals may occur.
6. Plaster should be well-molded otherwise abnormal pressure causes ulcerations and proper correction cannot be achieved. Sometimes loosening of plaster cast takes place.
7. Toes should be well exposed to visualize blood circulation.
8. Usually plaster casts are changed at weekly intervals except in the very early age where plaster can be changed at an interval of 5 days.
9. Care should be taken that there should be no over crowding of the toes which may lead to ulceration of the toes.

10. Proper correction should be adopted before tenotomy like 60° to 70° of abduction and 0° to 5° of dorsiflexion, because the amount of abduction achieved before and after tenotomy always remains the same. The presumption that the abduction angle will increase after tenotomy is wrong. After tenotomy the dorsiflexion should be 15° to 20° and abduction should be 60° to 70°.
11. Orthotic shoes are of utmost importance as any negligence of footwear may affect result of the treatment.
12. Proper massage and physiotherapy including exercises to facilitate dorsiflexion and abduction of the foot should be advocated.
13. A long follow-up at frequent intervals is mandatory to detect the recurrence of deformity at an earliest.

Derotation Around Talus

Deformities in clubfoot are not in a single plane; rather they are in a multiaxial plane; thus, deformities are corrected together. First, the supination of forefoot is done. Since the calcaneopedal block does not allow correction of deformity in pronated forefoot, thus supination is of utmost importance to eliminate the calcaneopedal block. The calcaneo-forefoot deformity is gradually corrected by abduction of the foot **(Figs. 8.9A to E)**.

Adduction of Forefoot

Adduction of forefoot on hindfoot is a horizontal plane deformity, which is to be observed from the plantar surface. Usually the deformity is corrected by abducting the forefoot gradually until it reaches 60° to 70° of abduction. The correction of this deformity is necessary for correction of equinus deformity **(Figs. 8.10A to E)**.

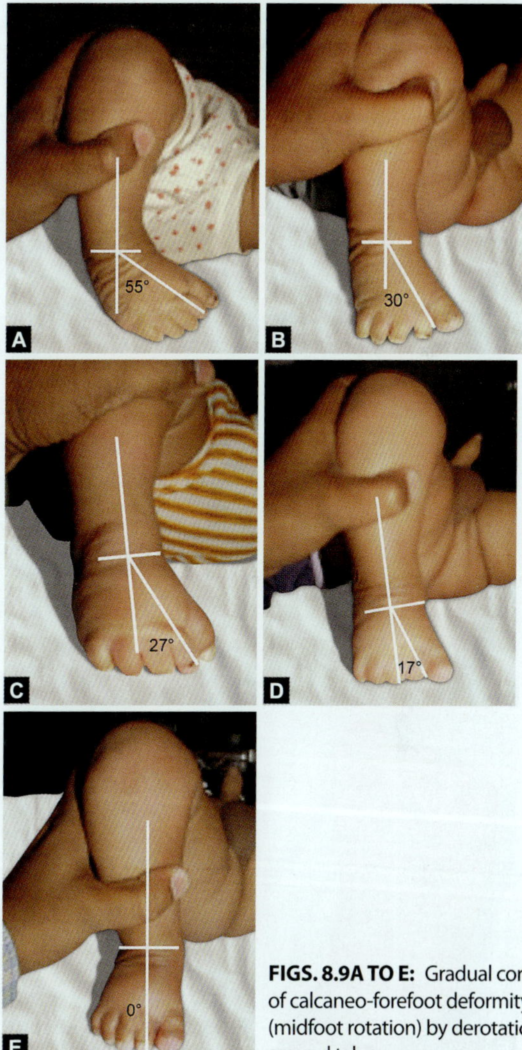

FIGS. 8.9A TO E: Gradual correction of calcaneo-forefoot deformity (midfoot rotation) by derotation around talus

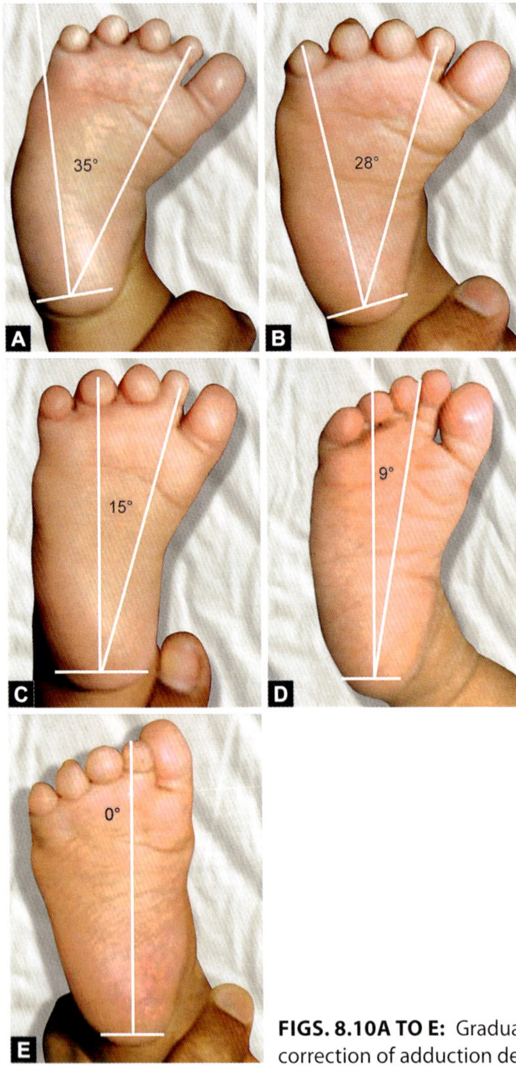

FIGS. 8.10A TO E: Gradual correction of adduction deformity

Varus Heel

Varus deformity of the heel is a frontal plane deformity to be viewed from back. Varus deformity is caused by inversion and internal rotation of calcaneus, which is the main culprit for all deformities, which sometimes reaches up to 75° to 90°. As soon as forefoot and hindfoot deformities are corrected, varus deformity is gradually corrected. The abduction of forefoot and midfoot causes abduction of calcaneum, which gradually corrects the varus deformity **(Figs. 8.11A to E)**.

Equinus Foot

Equinus deformity is caused by contracture of tendo-Achilles and contracture of posterior capsule. This deformity is corrected in the last. Percutaneous tendo-Achilles tenotomy is needed in most of the cases and 60° to 70° of abduction is mandatory before performing tendo-Achilles tenotomy. The foot is kept in 60° to 70° abduction and 15° to 20° dorsiflexion after tenotomy **(Figs. 8.12A to E)**.

Radiological Evaluation after Serial Plaster Casts

Radiographic assessment of clubfoot is important during serial plasters done for correction of clubfoot deformity. The radiographs are taken in anteroposterior standing view of 24° cephalad angulation and in lateral standing view. The anteroposterior and lateral view demonstrates talo-calcaneal, talo-first metatarsal and calcaneo-fifth metatarsal angle.

Talo-calcaneal angle: The normal range of talo-calcaneal angle is 13°–29° (mean angle is 20°) but in the clubfoot the anterior portion of calcaneus lies beneath the head of talus

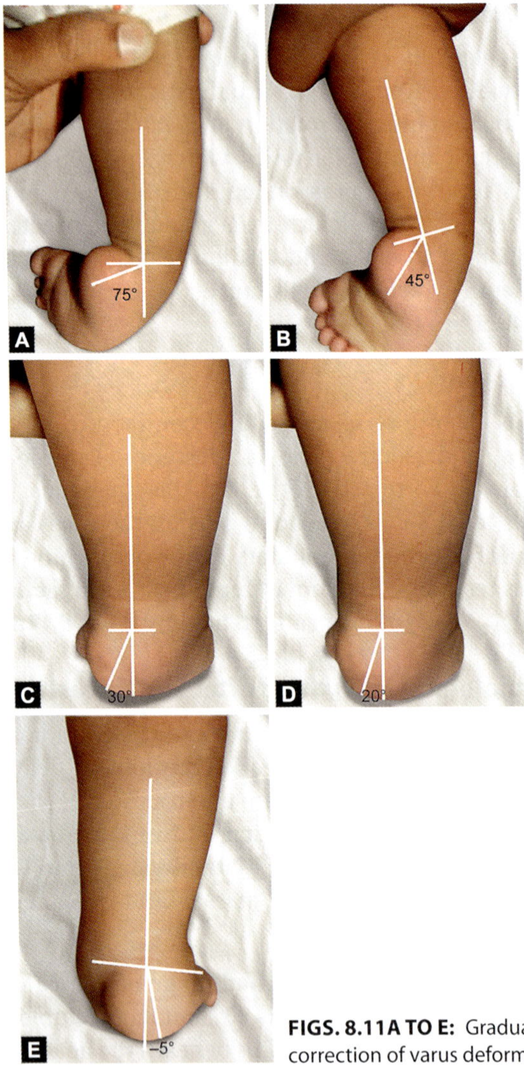

FIGS. 8.11A TO E: Gradual correction of varus deformity

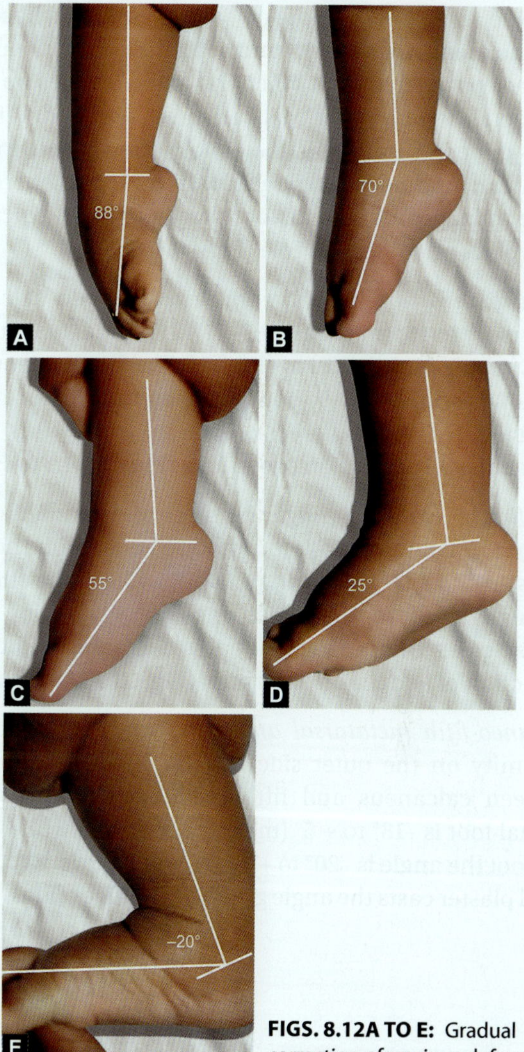

FIGS. 8.12A TO E: Gradual correction of equinus deformity

thus, the angle between the calcaneus and talus becomes less (the mean angle is 15°) and sometimes calcaneus and talus are parallel to each other and angle reaches up to 4°. As soon as serial plaster casts are given and abduction of foot is done in supination, the cuboid bone gives thrust to the calcaneus thus the angle gradually increases, therefore, in the management of clubfoot deformity; talo-calcaneal angle plays an important role **(Figs. 8.13A to E)**.

Talo-calcaneal angle in lateral view: The talo-calcaneal angle is 17° to 46° (mean angle is 31°) in normal foot and 10° to 34° (mean angle is 23°) in clubfoot. The foot is in equinus position in clubfoot. As soon as the equinus deformity is corrected, the angle increases even up to 46°. This angle represents the correction of equinus **(Figs. 8.14A to E)**.

Talo-first metatarsal angle: It indicates adduction of forefoot in comparison to hindfoot. The angle in normal foot is –20° to + 11° (mean angle is –3°) while in the clubfoot the angle is –10° to +33° (mean angle is +3°). During serial plaster casts this angle gradually decreases indicating correction of adduction deformity **(Figs. 8.15A to E)**.

Calcaneo-fifth metatarsal angle: It represents adduction deformity on the outer side of foot. The angle is taken between calcaneus and fifth metatarsal. The angle in normal foot is –18° to + 5° (mean angle is –3°) while in the clubfoot the angle is –20° to +20° (mean angle is –4°). In the serial plaster casts the angle gradually reduces **(Figs. 8.16A to E)**.

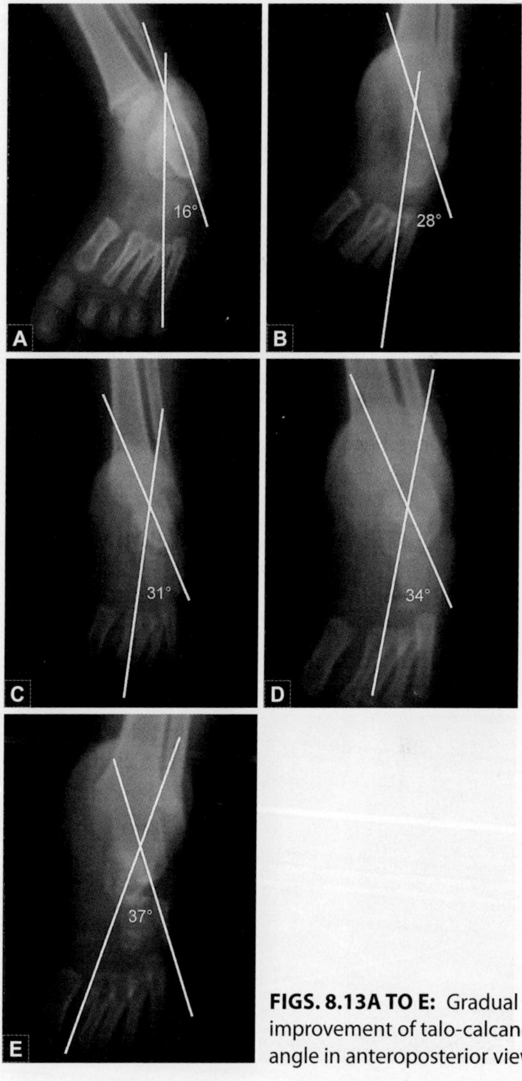

FIGS. 8.13A TO E: Gradual improvement of talo-calcaneal angle in anteroposterior view

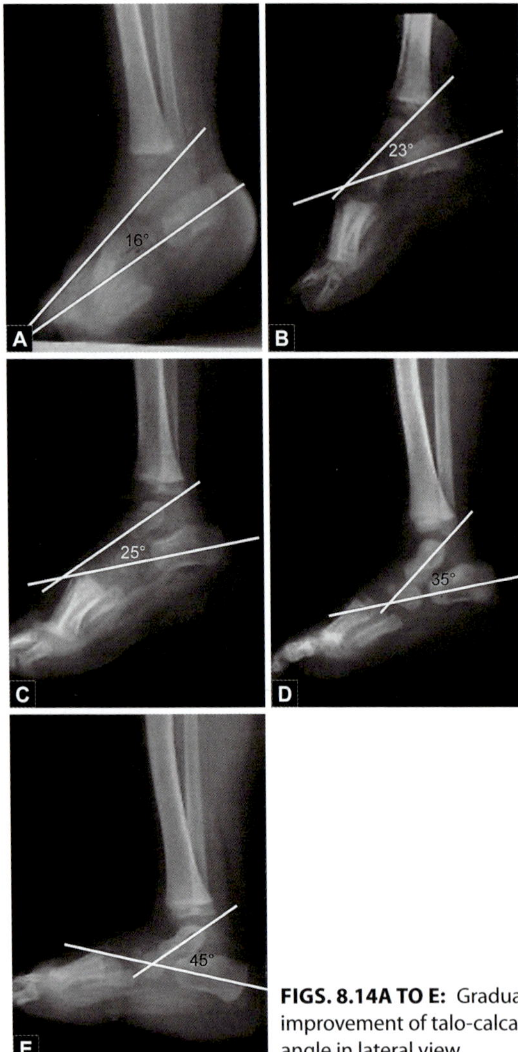

FIGS. 8.14A TO E: Gradual improvement of talo-calcaneal angle in lateral view

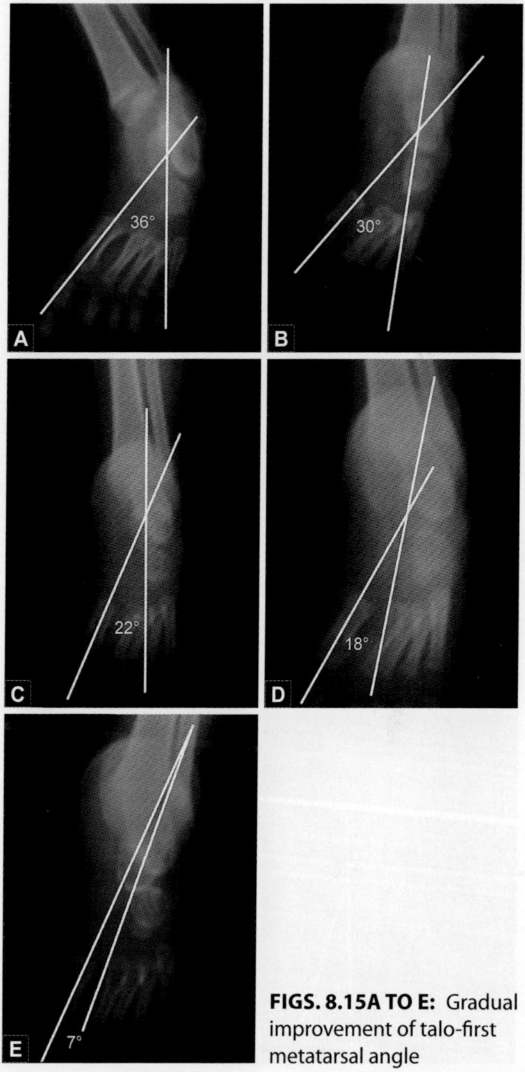

FIGS. 8.15A TO E: Gradual improvement of talo-first metatarsal angle

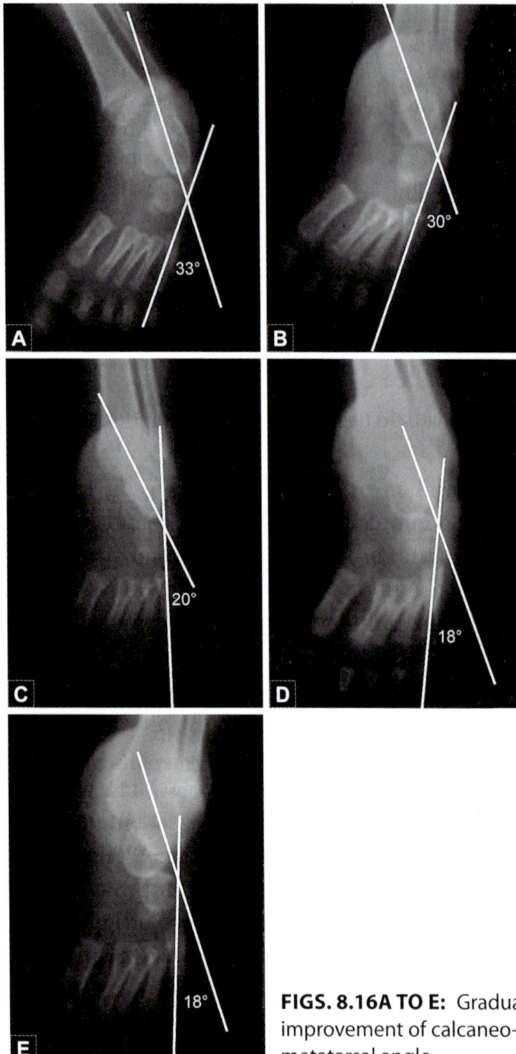

FIGS. 8.16A TO E: Gradual improvement of calcaneo-fifth metatarsal angle

Case 1: Congenital Clubfoot (0–1 year)

A 3-month-old male child with congenital clubfoot (right side) was treated by manipulation and plaster cast application by Ponseti technique. Four plaster casts were required for correction of cavus, adduction and varus deformity. After correcting these deformities percutaneous tendo-Achilles tenotomy was performed and last plaster cast was given in full correction of equinus for 3 weeks **(Figs. 8.17A to H)**.

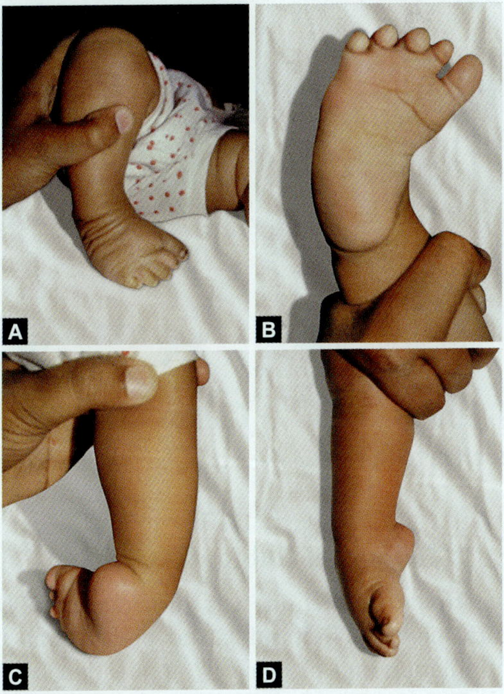

FIGS. 8.17A TO D: Pretreatment appearane of clubfoot showing midfoot rotation, adduction, varus and equinus

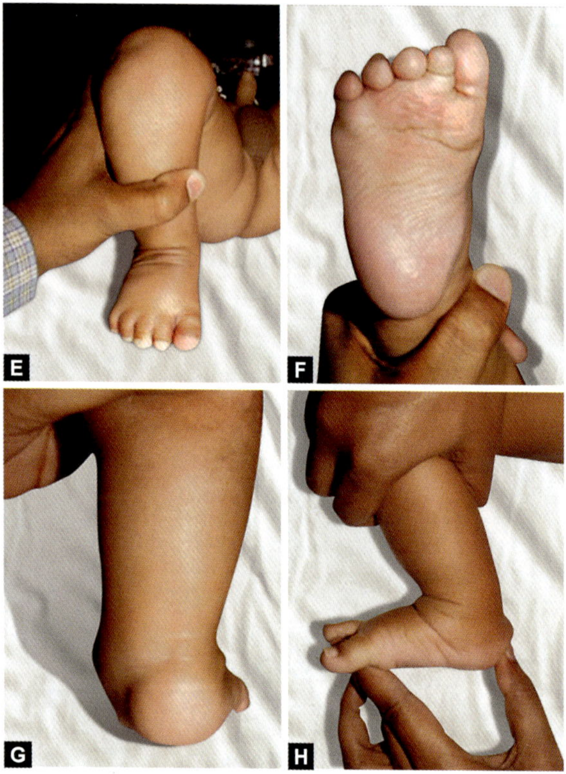

FIGS. 8.17E TO H: Final appearance of the foot after treatment

Case 2: Congenital Clubfoot (1–2 years)

A 1½-year-old male child was brought to OPD with congenital clubfoot (left side). The patient was treated by manipulation and plaster cast application by Ponseti method. Deformities of clubfoot were corrected in due course of time; five plaster casts were required to correct all deformities except equinus. Finally, percutaneous tendo-Achilles tenotomy was performed and sixth plaster cast was applied for 3 weeks **(Figs. 8.18A to H)**.

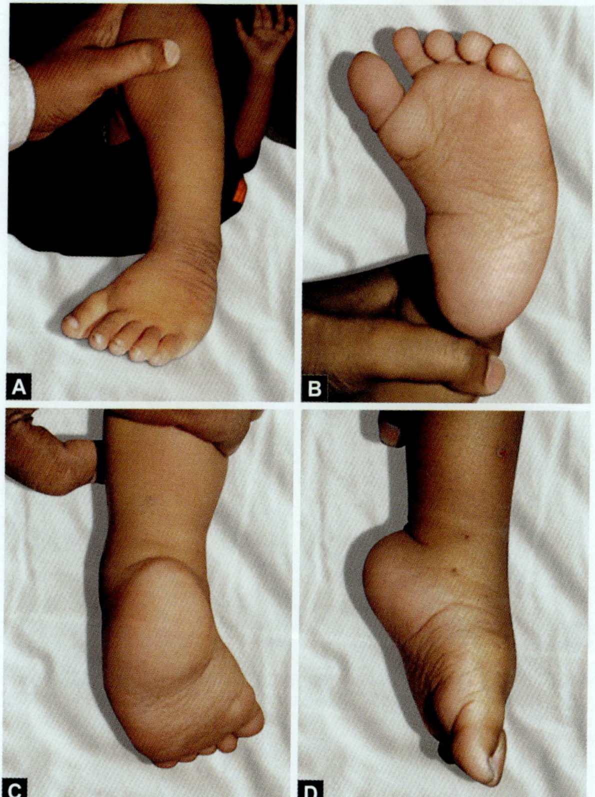

FIGS. 8.18A TO D: Pretreatment appearance of clubfoot showing midfoot rotation, adduction, varus and equinus

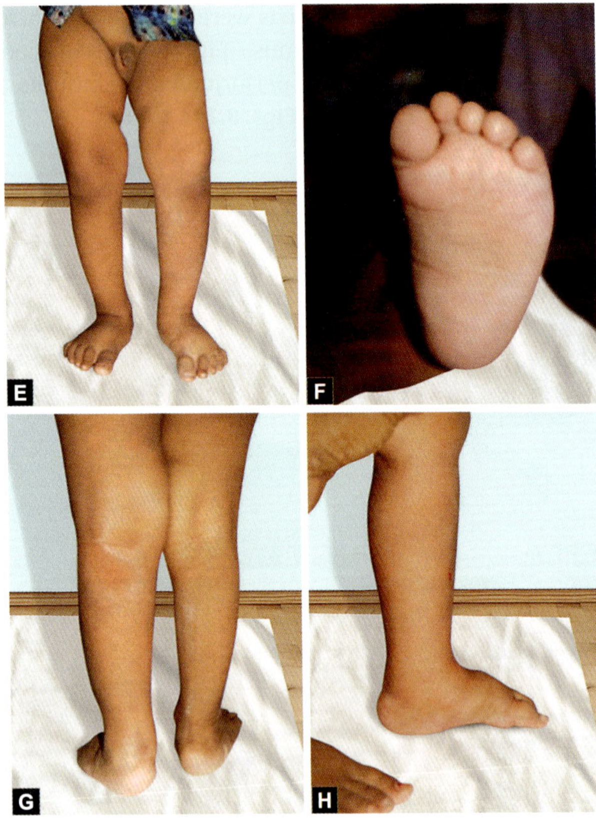

FIGS. 8.18E TO H: Final appearance of the foot after treatment

CHAPTER 9

Neglected Clubfoot

It is difficult to define neglected clubfoot. Though we worked out 9 months as the demarcating line for labelling as "Neglected Clubfoot", Stahele in his monograph on Ponseti technique has kept 2 years as demarcating line for Neglected Clubfoot from management point of view. Neglect may occur in proper selection of corrective modes and measures, proper conduction of treatment procedure, proper post-corrective physiotherapy and orthotic fittings, proper follow-ups etc. Each of the above can lead to the picture of neglected clubfoot **(Fig. 9.1** and **Flowchart 9.1)**.

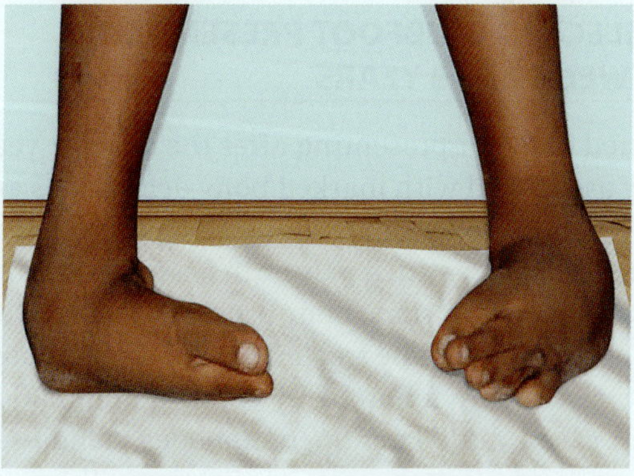

FIG. 9.1: Neglected clubfoot

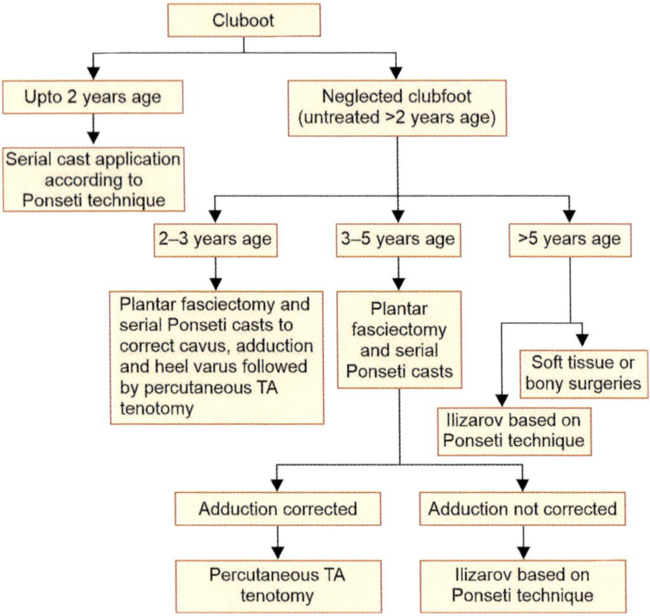

FLOWCHART 9.1: Algorithm of treatment of clubfoot

NEGLECTED CLUBFOOT PRESENTING BETWEEN 2 TO 3 YEARS

Neglected clubfoot presenting after the age of 2 years are usually associated with marked bony deformities and soft tissue contractures. In most of these cases surgery is the treatment of choice which may be in form of posteromedial soft tissue release or some bony procedures. But, we found that most of them can be treated initially by percutaneous plantar fasciotomy followed by serial manipulation and plaster casts and later percutaneous tendo-Achilles tenotomy and plaster cast application. There are so many contracted tissues but basic deforming forces are contracture of plantar fascia that causes pronation of forefoot in relation to midfoot and hindfoot, which leads to cavus deformity and contracture of tendo-Achilles which further leads to equinus deformity. These neglected feet are treated by percutaneous plantar fasciotomy under local anaesthesia followed by weekly manipulation and plaster cast application by Ponseti method. After achieving correction of adduction and cavus deformity, a second stage percutaneous tendo-Achilles tenotomy is performed under local anaesthesia and final plaster cast is applied for three weeks in 10–20° dorsiflexion at ankle and 50–70° abduction of foot.

Method

First Stage

Percutaneous plantar fasciotomy is performed under local anaesthesia after taking proper aseptic precautions, as an outdoor procedure. A 15 number surgical blade is inserted with its cutting edge turned backward on the anteromedial aspect of heel (about two fingers below and 0.5 cm in front of the tip of the medial malleolus). The blade is then gradually tilted upward to reach the under surface of the calcaneum. When bony resistance is felt the cutting edge of the blade is gradually tilted to 90° of the planter surface of the heel **(Fig. 9.2)**. Simultaneously, by holding the foot at about mid and forefoot junction by other hand, it is gradually taken to the corrected position as far as possible. In this manoeuvre one can feel and hear the cutting of tight ligaments and other contracted soft tissues which yield to a variable extent. By cautiously manipulating the scalpel blade under the calcaneum, any other tight tissues (ligament, tendon,

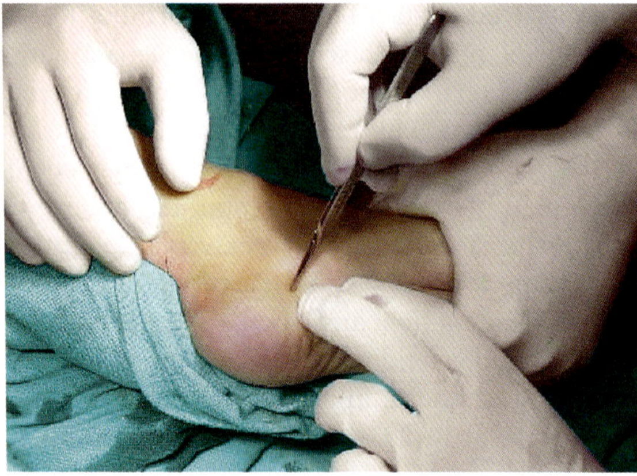

FIG. 9.2: Percutaneous plantar fasciotomy

muscle origins, fibrous tissue) can be further cut. The main precaution to be taken in this procedure is to avoid any possible damage to the neurovascular bundle by always remaining close to the bone and never turning the cutting edge of the blade to the medial side. The blade is withdrawn and the punctured wound is pressed to secure haemostasis.

Thereafter, manipulation is started by Ponseti technique and above knee plaster cast is applied. The patient is reviewed weekly for manipulation and plaster cast reapplication till 50°–70° abduction of foot is achieved. Number of plaster casts may vary due to varying degree of contractures and maturity of ligaments.

Second Stage

After attaining adequate correction of adduction and cavus deformity, second stage percutaneous tendo-Achilles tenotomy is done. It is performed under local anaesthesia after taking proper aseptic precautions, as an outdoor procedure. Tendon is palpated 1–2 cm above its insertion and a small amount of 2% Xylocaine is infiltrated near the tendon. A 15 number blade is inserted with its cutting edge facing downward anterior to the tendon and dorsiflexion is performed by other hand, now the cutting edge is turned 90° posteriorly cutting the tight tendon. A pop is felt and immediate 10–20° dorsiflexion is achieved. Haemostasis is achieved by pressure and sterile dressing pad applied. Post-tenotomy plaster cast is applied with foot in 50–70° abduction and 10–20° dorsiflexion. Plaster cast is kept for 3 weeks. After 3 weeks cast is removed; bracing and regular physiotherapy is started.

Case 1

A 2-year and 7-month-old male child was brought to OPD with neglected clubfoot (right side). The patient was initially treated by percutaneous plantar fasciotomy under local anaesthesia followed by manipulation and weekly plaster casts by Ponseti technique. Total six plaster casts were required to correct cavus and adduction deformity. In second stage percutaneous tendo-Achilles tenotomy was performed under local anaesthesia followed by plaster cast for 21 days in corrected position **(Fig. 9.3)**.

NEGLECTED CLUBFOOT PRESENTING BETWEEN 3 TO 5 YEARS

From treatment point of view, children between the age of 3 to 5 years present some difficulties due to relative maturity of soft tissues, ligaments and bones of foot. Therefore, treatment adopted is a middle path protocol. The treatment begins with percutaneous plantar fasciotomy followed by

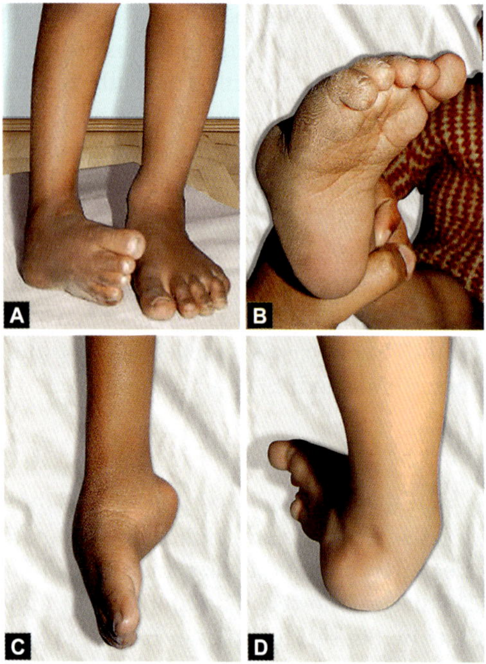

FIGS. 9.3A TO D: Pre-treatment photographs

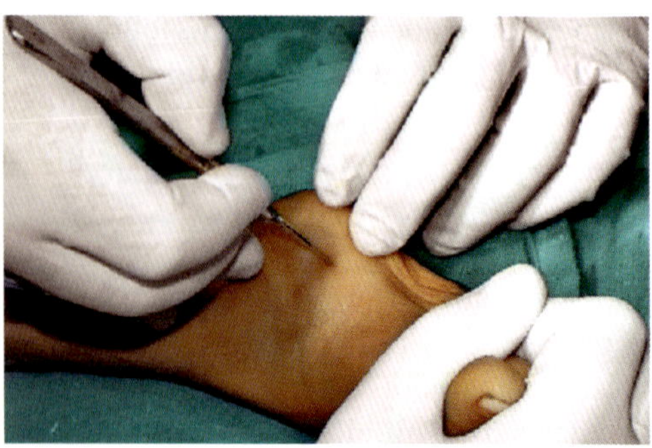

FIG. 9.3E: Percutaneous plantar fasciotomy

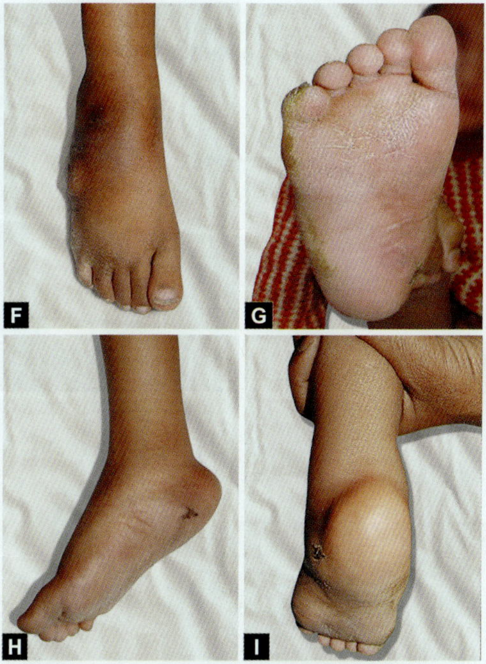

FIGS. 9.3F TO I: After plantar fasciotomy and serial plaster cast

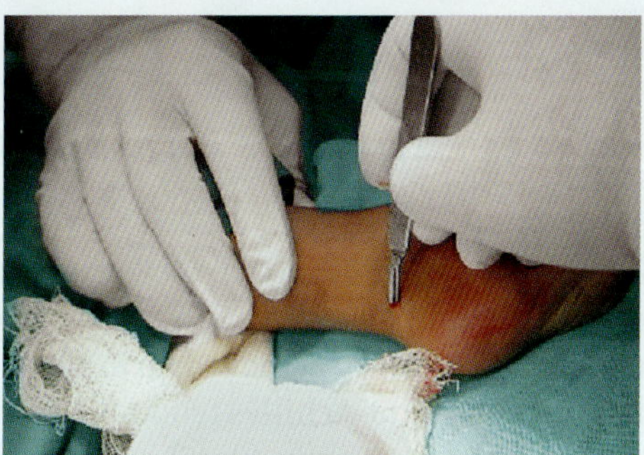

FIG. 9.3J: Percutaneous TA tenotomy

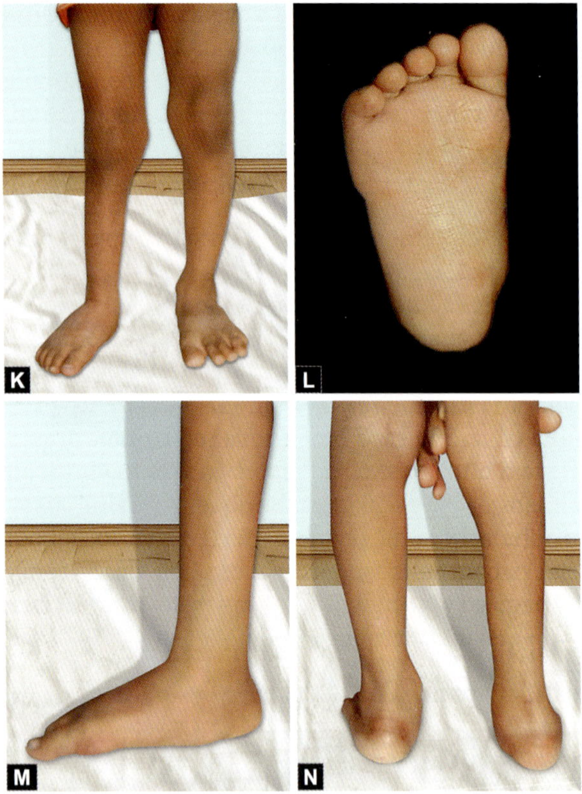

FIGS. 9.3K TO N: Final photographs after plantar fasciotomy and tendo-Achilles tenotomy

manipulation and serial Ponseti cast to correct adduction deformity. If adduction deformity can be corrected easily and abduction of foot can be achieved up to 30–40°, second stage percutaneous tendo-Achilles tenotomy is performed and final plaster cast is given in 10–15° of dorsiflexion and 30–40° of abduction for 3 weeks.

It is inevitable to expect problems in achieving correction of adduction deformity because of stiffness of foot. Therefore, if it is not possible to achieve 30°- 40° of abduction after serial plaster casts at weekly interval, Ilizarov fixator should be applied and gradual distraction is performed to correct adduction deformity followed by correction of equinus deformity after performing tendo-Achilles tenotomy.

Case 2

A 5-year-old boy with neglected bilateral congenital clubfoot was treated by percutaneous plantar fasciotomy under local anaesthesia followed by manipulation and plaster casts by Ponseti technique. In second stage percutaneous tendo-Achilles tenotomy was performed under local anaesthesia and final plaster cast was given for 21 days. Correction was achieved on left side but right side still had adduction deformity. For correction of adduction deformity Ilizarov fixator was applied and finally deformity was corrected **(Figs. 9.4A to O)**.

NEGLECTED CLUBFOOT PRESENTING AFTER 5 YEARS OF AGE

1. Ilizarov technique based on Ponseti principle
2. Soft tissue and bony surgeries

ILIZAROV TECHNIQUE BASED ON PONSETI PRINCIPLE

This procedure of controlled fractional distraction lengthens the contracted tissues promoting histogenesis which also controls the magnitude of correction of the

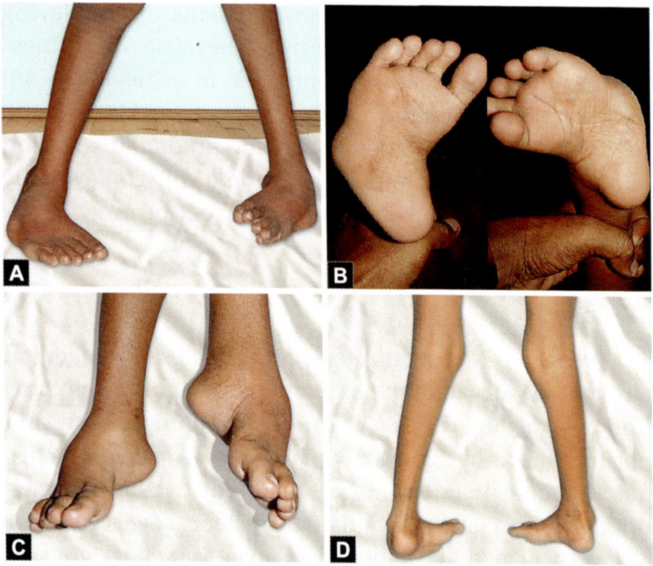

FIGS. 9.4A TO D: Pretreatment photographs of neglected clubfoot showing midfoot rotation, adduction, equinus and varus

component deformities depending upon the severity. However, procedures like Steindler's plantar fasciotomy and tendo-Achilles lengthening are essential to avoid under correction and complications. One must be cautious at every step to watch for distal ischaemia of the toes and pin tract infection. The attendants and patients proper compliance is essential for the success of these procedures.

Role of Ilizarov fixator for correction of clubfoot is well described by Bradish (2000) up to the age of 11 years but with fixation of calcaneum with 2 wires. Lamm et al (2006) also described use of external fixator in clubfoot.

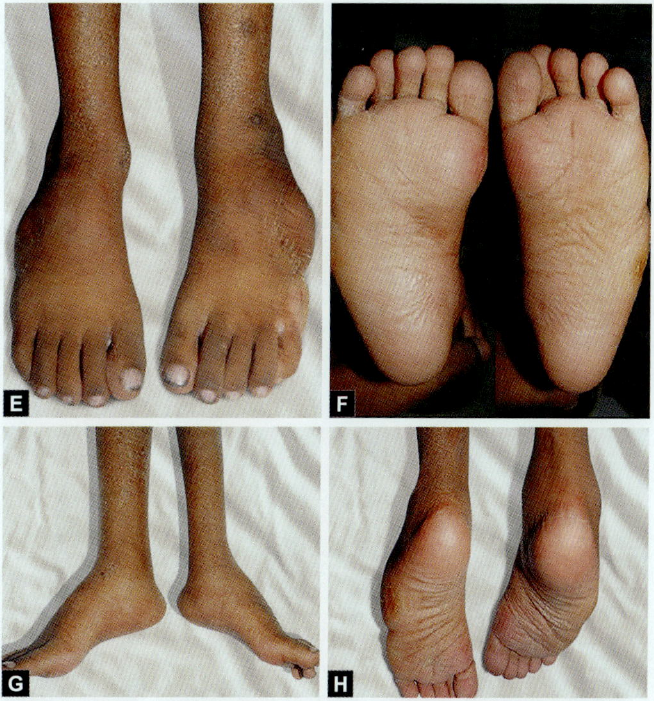

FIGS. 9.4E TO H: After plantar fasciotomy and serial plaster cast

After 5 years of age, we treat rigid and neglected clubfoot by Ilizarov fixator based on Ponseti principles.

Correction of neglected clubfoot presenting after 5 years of age by Ilizarov technique based on Ponseti principle:

A. Frame Construction
B. Steps of Deformity Correction
C. Post Removal Bracing

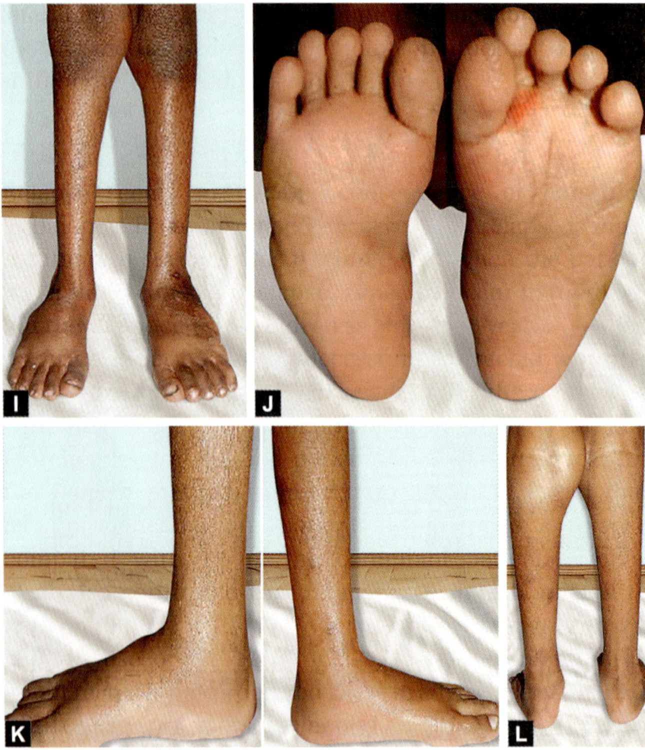

FIGS. 9.4I TO L: After TA tenotomy and serial plaster cast

Frame Construction

For frame construction one must be very particular with the site of K-wires. For proper positioning of K-wires use of image intensifier is inevitable.

Site of K-wires

1. *Proximal tibial wires*: Two K-wires (1.8 mm) are inserted at the junction of upper and middle-third of tibia.

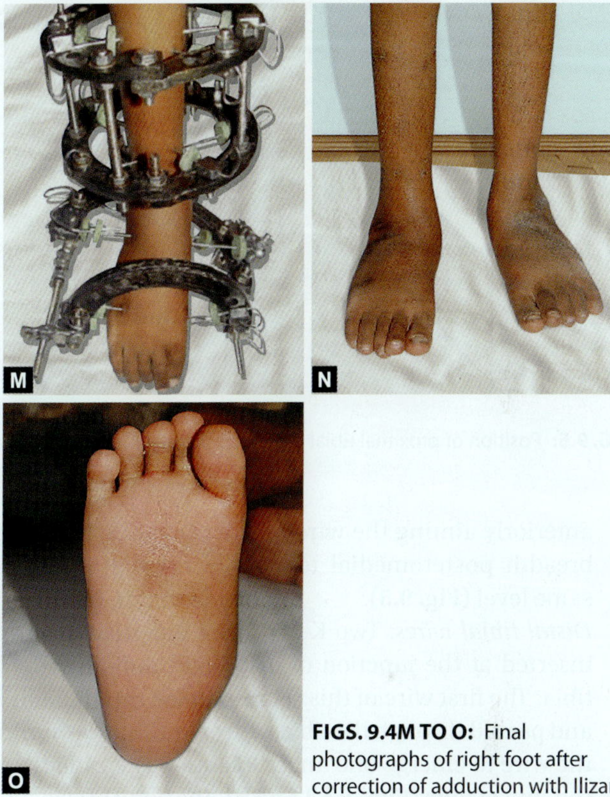

FIGS. 9.4M TO O: Final photographs of right foot after correction of adduction with Ilizaro

The first wire is inserted at about one fingerbreadth lateral and behind the shin of tibia with an inclination of the wire aiming to emerge at the same level just anterior to the medial border. Second wire is inserted about one fingerbreadth anterior to the palpable anterior border of fibula at a point about 5 mm (thickness of ring 4 mm) below the level of first wire and with an inclination

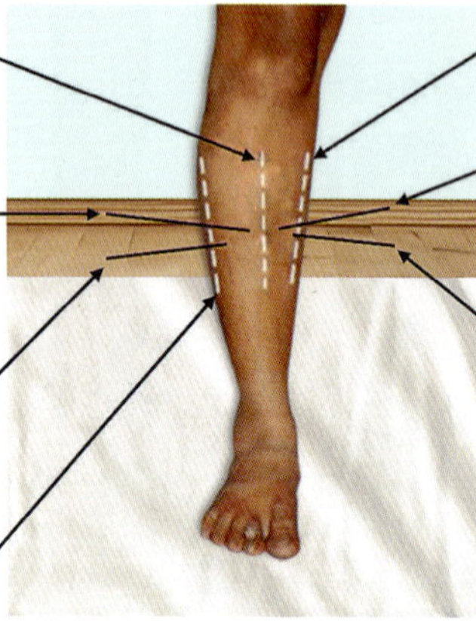

FIG. 9.5: Position of proximal tibial wires

anteriorly aiming the wire to emerge about one finger breadth posteromedial to shin of tibia at about the same level **(Fig. 9.5)**.

2. *Distal tibial wires*: Two K-wires (1.8 mm diameter) are inserted at the junction of distal and middle-third of tibia. The first wire of this set is inserted through fibula and passed through the tibia with an inclination aiming the wire to emerge one fingerbreadth posteromedial to the shin of tibia **(Figs. 9.6A and B)**. The point of selection for inserting the second wire should be done cautiously. The space between the anterior border of tibia and fibula is divided into three equal zones. The anterior zone contains neurovascular structures and tendons. The middle zone is more or less safe containing mostly the muscular part **(Fig. 9.6A)**. At about 5 mm (note that the thickness of ring 4 mm) below the level of the first wire, the second wire is inserted through the safe corridor of

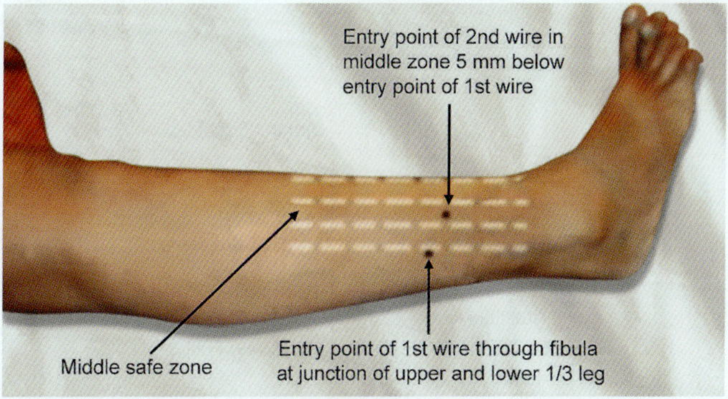

FIG. 9.6A: Entry point of distal tibial wires

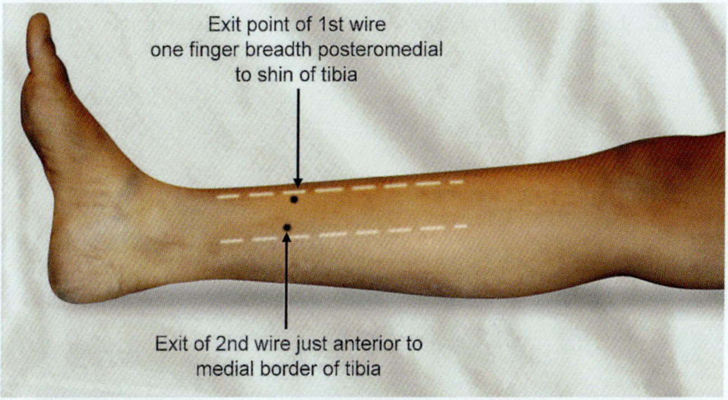

FIG. 9.6B: Exit point of 1st and 2nd wire

middle zone into the tibia with an inclination to emerge just anterior to the medial border of tibia **(Figs. 9.6A to C)**. One should be careful to avoid piercing of the great saphenous vein which crosses the medial border of tibia about 5 fingerbreadths above medial malleolus in anteroposterior direction **(Fig. 9.6D)**.

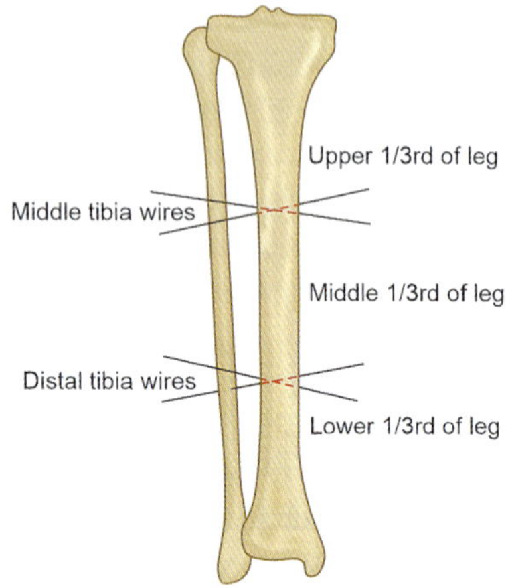

FIG. 9.6C: Position of wires for proximal and distal tibial rings

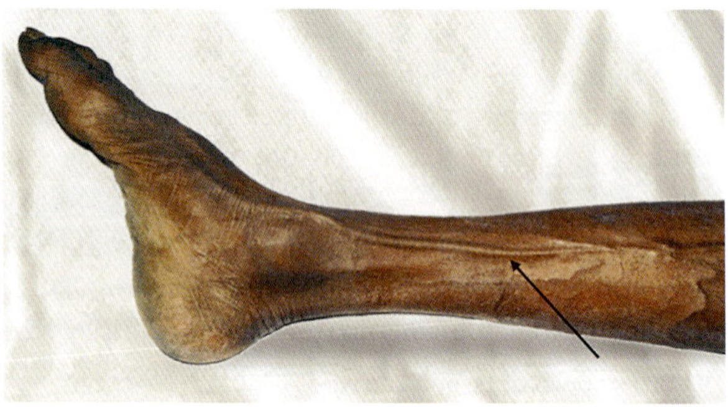

FIG. 9.6D: Position of great saphenous vein

3. *Midfoot talar wires*: Now, put two rings in the foot—one in the midfoot and another in the forefoot. The two wires holding the midfoot ring pass through the head of the talus **(Figs. 9.7A and B)**.

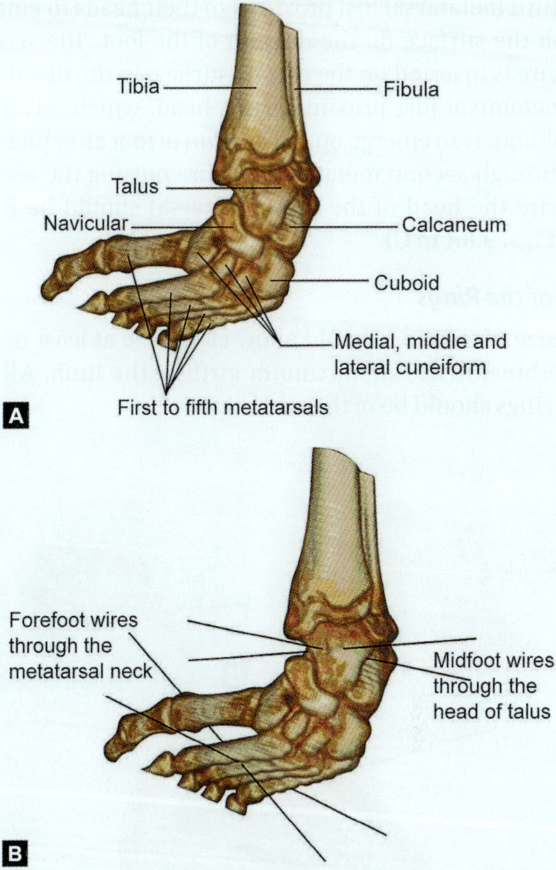

FIGS. 9.7A AND B: Anatomy of clubfoot and position of wires

4. *Forefoot metatarsal wires*: In the forefoot, the first wire is inserted from the outer side through the distal part of the fifth metatarsal between the head and neck and is advanced obliquely piercing the fifth, fourth and

third metatarsal just proximal to their heads to emerge on the surface on the dorsum of the foot. The second wire is inserted on the medial surface in the distal first metatarsal just proximal to its head, which advances obliquely to emerge on the dorsum of foot after piercing through second metatarsal. Before putting the second wire the head of the first metatarsal should be lifted **(Figs. 9.8A to C)**.

Size of the Rings

The size of the ring should allow clearance at least of two fingerbreadth at the maximum girth of the limb. All the four rings should be of the same size.

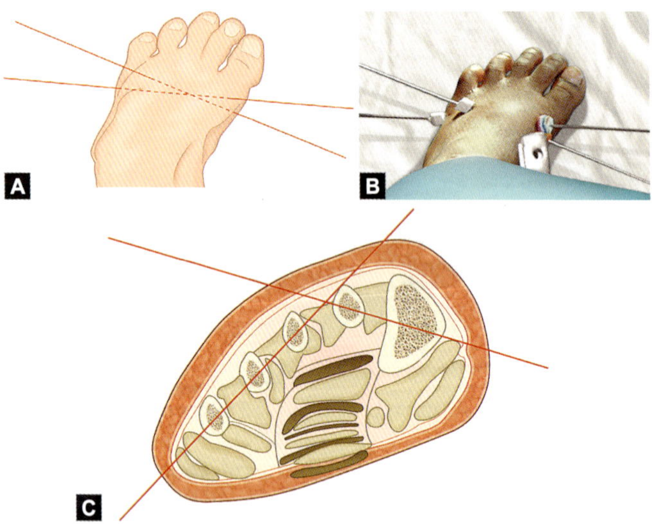

FIGS. 9.8A TO C: Position of K-wires in forefoot

Position of Rings

Proximal tibial ring: A full ring is placed approximately at the junction of upper third to middle third of the leg **(Fig. 9.9)**.

Distal tibial ring: A full ring is placed about 10–12 cm above the ankle joint, i.e. at about the junction of lower-third and middle third of leg **(Fig. 9.9)**.

Midfoot and forefoot rings: Two full rings are placed around the foot, one in midfoot region at the level of the head of talus and second at the level of metatarsal neck in forefoot region **(Fig. 9.9)**.

Steps of Deformity Correction

STEP 1: Correction of Pronation of Forefoot

For the correction of clubfoot by Ponseti principle—first the plantar fasciotomy, i.e Steindler's release is performed,

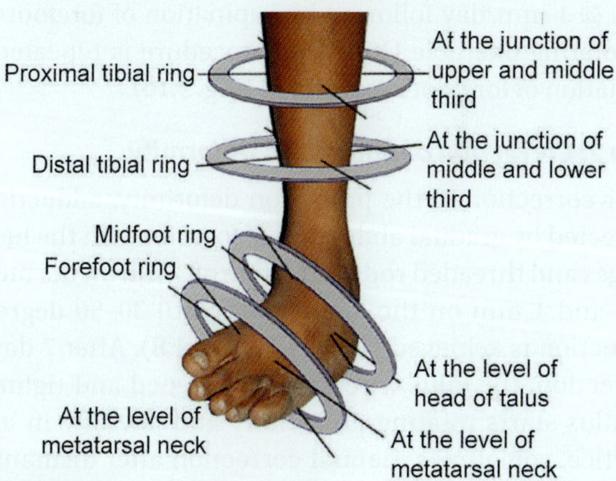

FIG. 9.9: Frame configuration

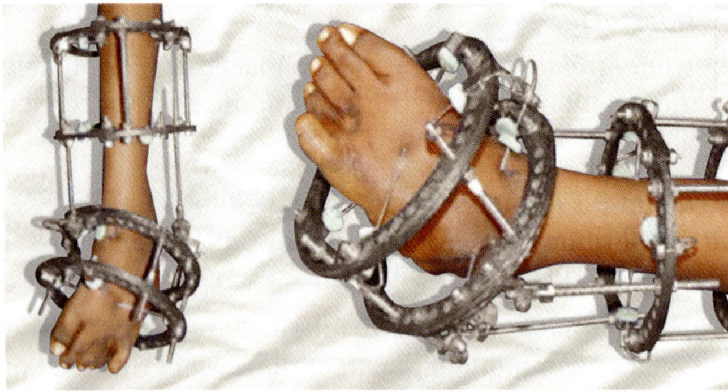

FIG. 9.10: (Distraction of foot, Supination of forefoot). Distraction between forefoot and midfoot is done with the help of threaded rods fixed to the rings at the rate of 1–3 mm/day followed by 10° of supination (by rotating one hole every third day)

followed by correction of the forefoot pronation by gradual distraction between midfoot and forefoot ring for 3–5 days @ 1 mm/day followed by supination of forefoot ring by rotating one hole (10°). This procedure is repeated till pronation of forefoot is corrected **(Fig. 9.10)**.

Step 2: Correction of Adduction Deformity

After correction of the pronation deformity, adduction is corrected by gradual abduction of forefoot with the help of hinges and threaded rods at the rate of 3 mm on the medial side and 1 mm on the lateral side until 30–50 degree of abduction is achieved **(Figs. 9.11A and B)**. After 7 days of correction, the talus wire can be loosened and tightened as talus starts rotating posteriorly and laterally in ankle mortice, sometimes manual correction after dismantling

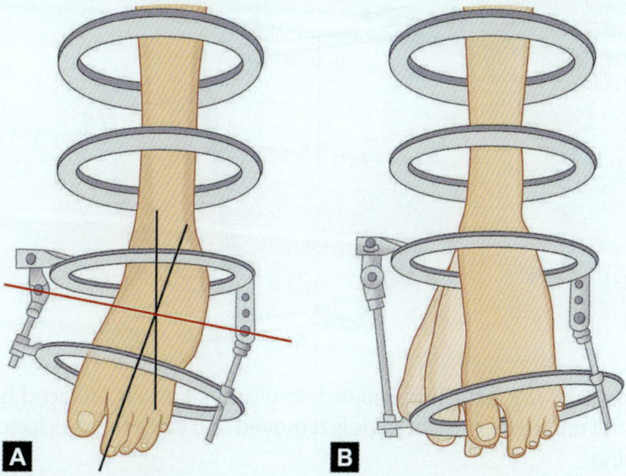

FIGS. 9.11A AND B: Gradual abduction of foot

of the threaded rods can be performed because corrections are not in single axis but in multiple axis.

Step 3: Correction of Equinus

After correcting adduction and pronation deformity of forefoot tendo-Achilles tenotomy is performed either by percutaneous two-stab method or percutaneous single stab method (ladder pattern tenotomy). The full ring of forefoot is replaced by half ring, full ring from head of talus is removed and a calcaneal half ring is applied with two 1.5 mm K-wires. Equinus is gradually corrected by distraction at the rate of 1 mm/day from day 7 (the day of tenotomy should be considered as day 1) **(Figs. 9.12A and B)**.

There are two methods of percutaneous tenotomy:

i. Single stab method
ii. Two stab method

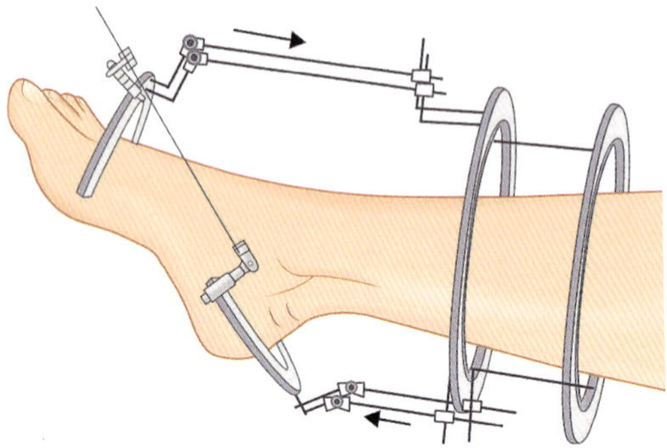

FIG. 9.12A: Correction of Equinus: forefoot full ring is replaced by half ring, full ring from head of talus is removed and calcaneous is fixed with half ring

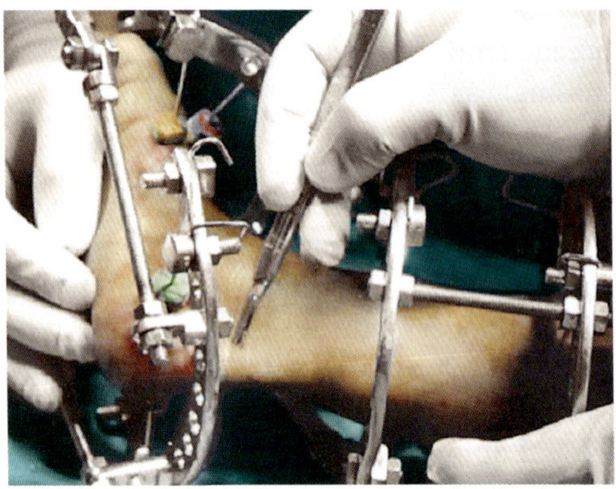

FIG. 9.12B: Single stab method of percutaneous tendo-Achilles tenotomy. All connecting threaded rods between foot and tibia are dismantled; percutaneous subtotal tendo-Achilles tenotomy is performed; frame is reassembled with 2 mm overriding of the tendo-Achilles cut ends by increasing the original equinus by 5°.

Percutaneous Method

Single Stab Method

One fingerbreadth above the insertion of tendo-Achilles, 2/3 to 3/4 of the girth of the Achilles tendon is severed by no. 15 B.P blade from anterior aspect **(Fig. 9.12B)**. The surgeon's another hand holds the forefoot in maximum possible dorsiflex position of the foot from the very beginning. As the tendo-Achilles gets severed, the dorsiflexed position of the foot increases with stretching of the weakened tendon. This gives a ladder pattern cut of the tendon even though the position of the blade has been kept static (**Figs 9.13A to G:** operative demonstration in a fresh cadaver for easy understanding). With further dorsiflexion tendoclasis occurs which can be heard and felt. Beyond this dorsiflexion is stopped and foot is replaced in the original equinus position with addition of 5° more to achieve about 2 mm overlapping of the tenotomized ends.

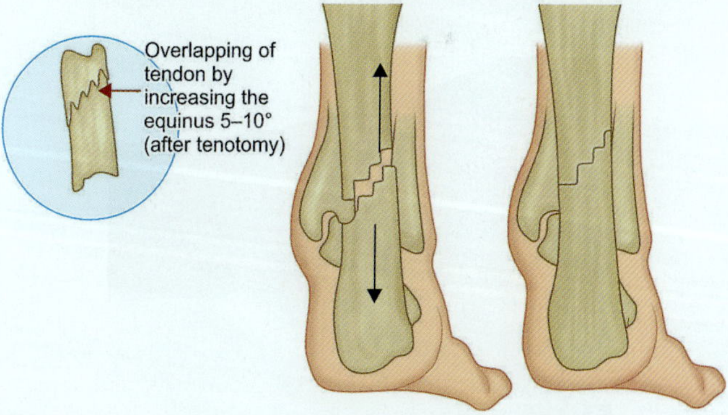

FIG. 9.13A: Showing ladder pattern tendo-Achilles tenotomy and lengthening

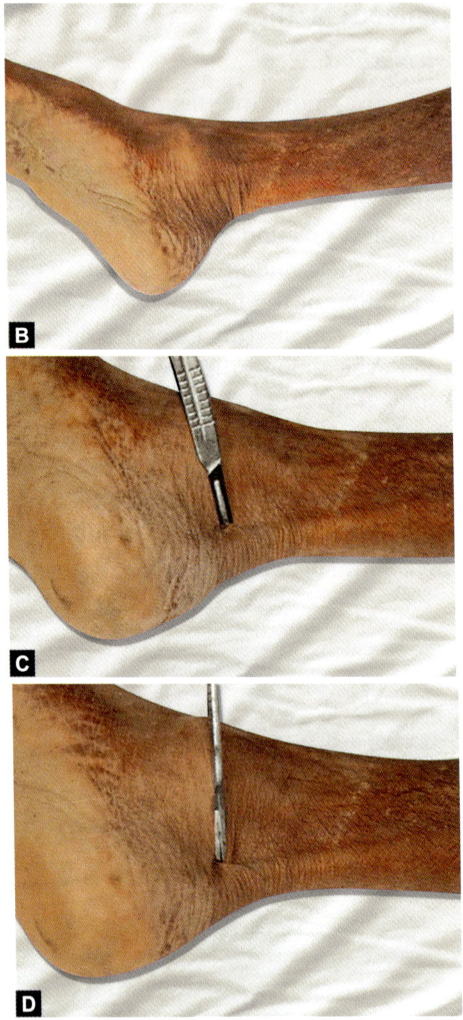

FIGS. 9.13B TO D: *Continued*

Continued

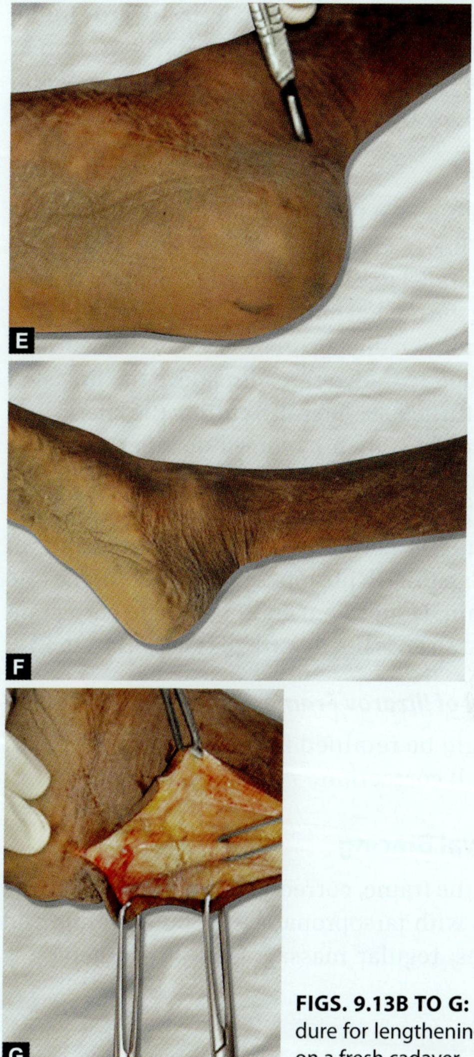

FIGS. 9.13B TO G: Single stab procedure for lengthening of tendo-Achilles on a fresh cadaver

This position is kept static for seven days. The remaining equinus deformity is corrected gradually by Ilizarov frame @ 1 mm/day from the 7th postoperative day (0.25 mm at 7 am, 11 am, 3 pm and 7 pm) (the day of tenotomy should be considered as day 1).

Two Stab Method

One fingerbreadth above the lowest attachment of tendo-Achilles, a no. 15 B.P. blade is introduced at the centre of the tendo-Achilles parallel to its fibres. The B.P. blade is turned medially cutting the medial half of the Achilles tendon. The B.P. blade is withdrawn and again inserted in the centre of the Achilles tendon two fingerbreadth above the first step and the blade is turned 90° laterally, cutting the lateral half of the Achilles tendon. Then by forced dorsiflexion of the foot lengthening of tendo-Achilles is achieved in continuity (medial-lateral Z lengthening in continuity). The remaining equinus deformity is corrected gradually at the rate of 1 mm per day from the 7th postoperative day, i.e. at the rate of 0.25 mm at 7 am, 11 am, 3 pm and 7 pm, night correction is avoided so that sleep is not disturbed **(Figs. 9.14A to E)**.

Step 4: Removal of Ilizarov Frame

The frame should be retained for a minimum period of 6 weeks after full correction.

Post Removal Bracing

After removing the frame, correction is maintained by the splints or boots with tarsopronator effect on the sole and corrective straps; regular massage and physiotherapy is started.

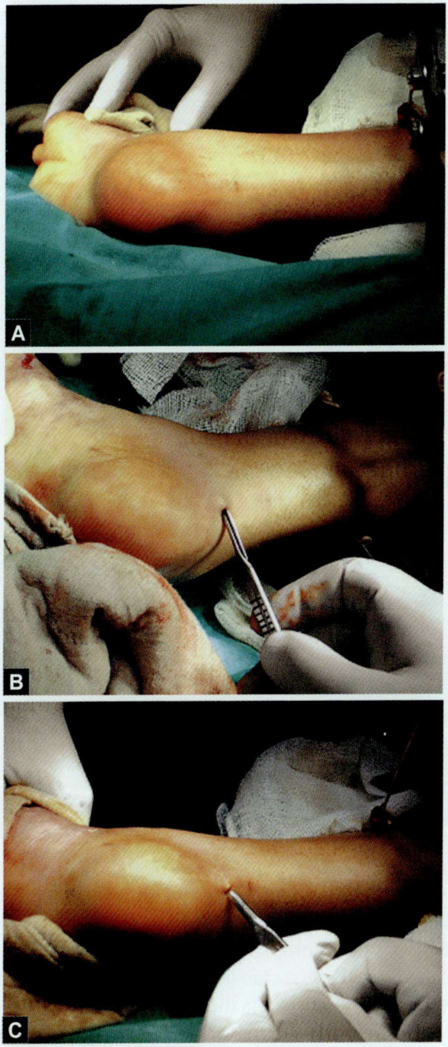

FIGS. 9.14A TO C: *Continued*

Continued

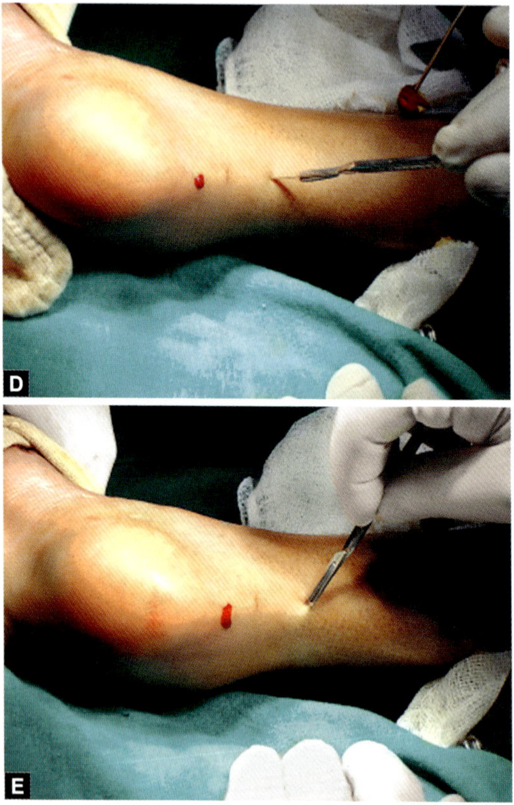

FIGS. 9.14A TO E: (A and B) A no. 15 B.P. blade is inserted in the centre of the tight heel cord at one fingerbreadth above the insertion of tendo-Achilles, (C) The blade is turned medially by 90° which cuts the medial-half of the heel cord, (D) The B.P. blade is again inserted two fingerbreadth above the first stab in the same way, (E) Then the blade is rotated by 90° laterally which cuts the lateral-half of the heel cord at that site. The blade is withdrawn. The foot is dorsiflexed. While performing percutaneous subtotal tenotomy, the B.P. blade should be handled carefully and piercing of posterior skin must be avoided

Case 3

A 17-year-old girl with neglected bilateral congenital clubfoot was treated by Ilizarov technique based on Ponseti principle. Gradually pronation of forefoot and adduction of foot were corrected followed by percutaneous tendo-Achilles tenotomy for equinus correction. Total duration of fixator for both foot was four and a half month. Result was good and she got painless normal looking functional foot **(Figs. 9.15A to E)**.

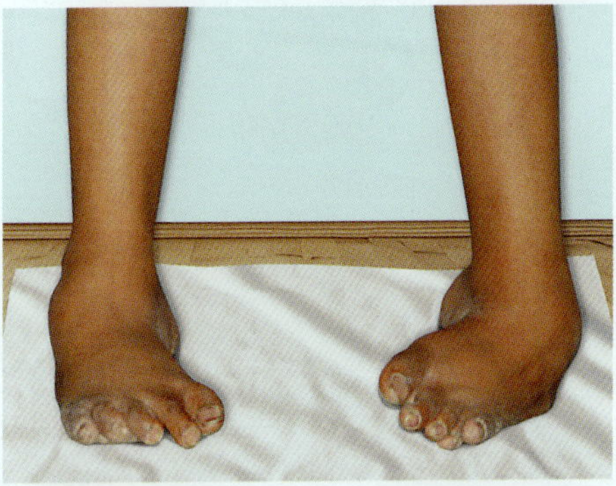

FIG. 9.15A: A 17-year-girl with congenital clubfoot

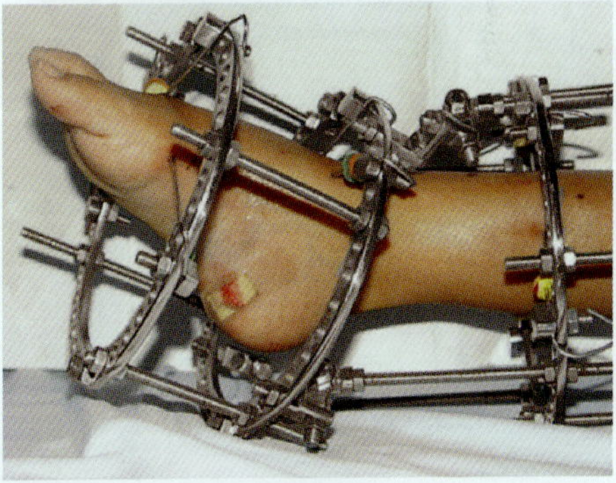

FIG. 9.15B: Forefoot supination

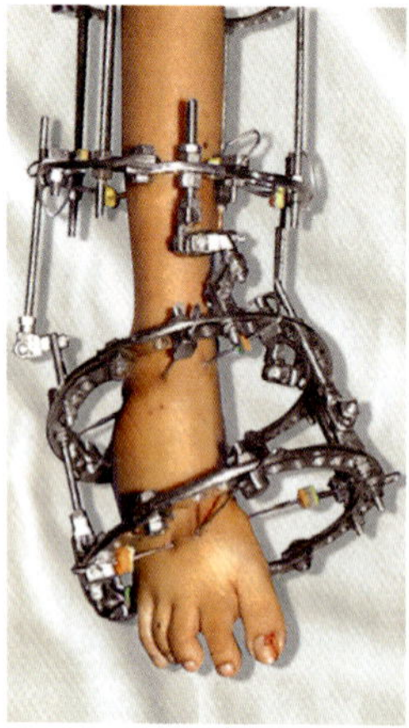

FIG. 9.15C: Correction of adduction

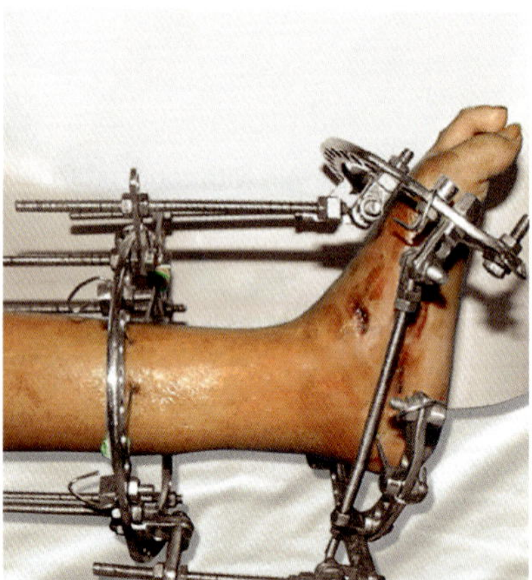

FIG. 9.15D: Correction of equinus

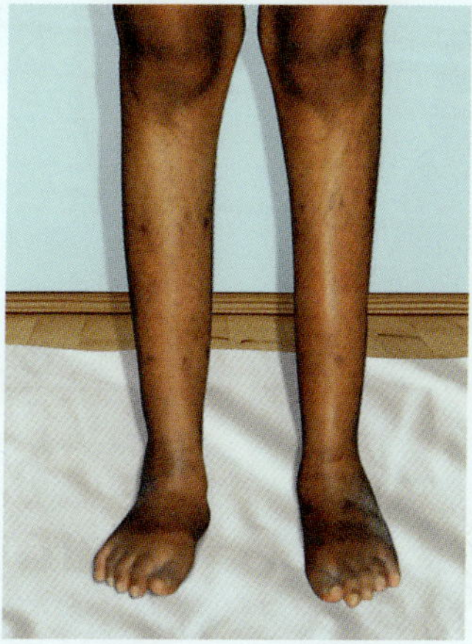

FIG. 9.15E: Final photograph of the same girl

FIGS 9.15A TO E: Serial photographs of a patient having B/L clubfoot deformity

Case 4

A 9-year-old girl with neglected congenital clubfoot (right side) was treated by Ilizarov technique based on Ponseti principle. Gradually the deformities were corrected followed by percutaneous tendo-Achilles tenotomy for equinus correction. Total duration of fixator for right foot was four months. Result is good and she got painless normal looking functional foot **(Figs. 9.16A to F)**.

Soft Tissue and Bony Surgeries

Open Method of Tendo-Achilles Lengthening

In cases of neglected clubfoot with severe equinus deformity open lengthening of tendo-Achilles is required.

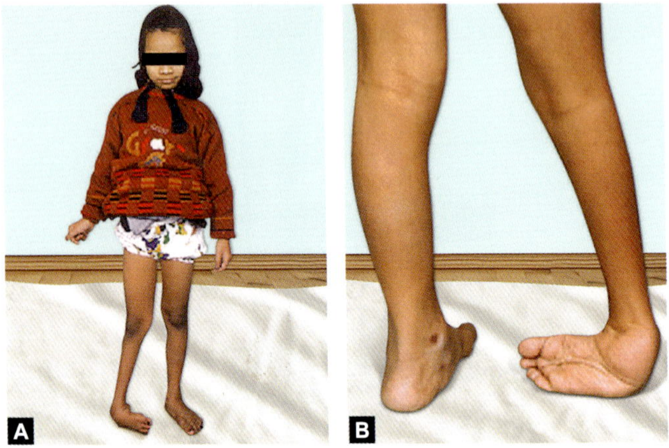

FIGS. 9.16A AND B: A 9-year-old girl with neglected clubfoot (right side)

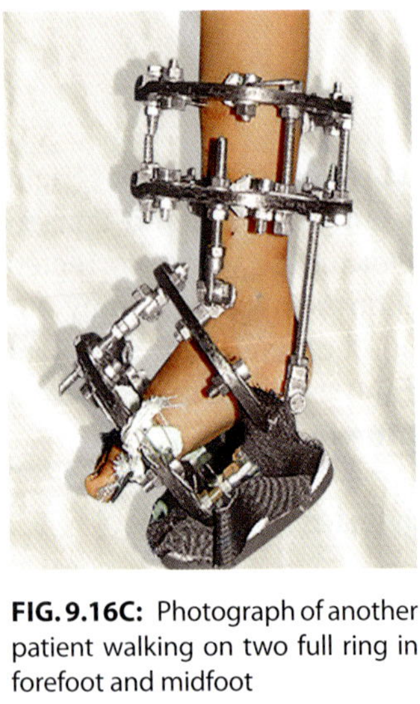

FIG. 9.16C: Photograph of another patient walking on two full ring in forefoot and midfoot

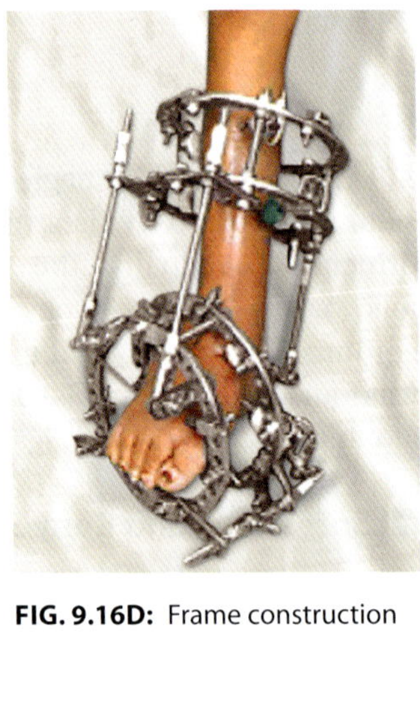

FIG. 9.16D: Frame construction

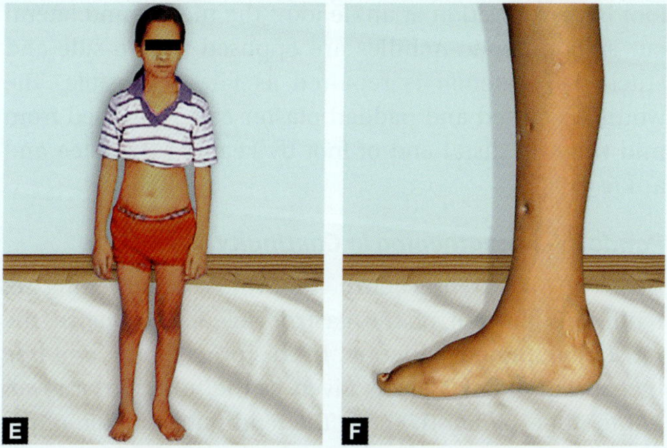

FIGS. 9.16E AND F: Final photograph of the same girl

Two common methods for open tendo-Achilles are described below.

Z-lengthening of Tendo-Achilles

A vertical incision is made starting from the insertion of the tendo-Achilles to the calcaneus to its musculotendinous junction parallel to the tendon on its medial side. The subcutaneous tissue is divided in the line of incision and retracted on both sides to expose the Achilles tendon covered with paratenon. After vertically dividing the paratenon, the contracted tendo-Achilles is cleared in its entire length and lengthened in a 'Z' fashion, the medial-half being released at its lower end from the calcaneus. The plantaris tendon is severed at its lower end. The fibroareolar tissue is cleared and the tight fibrous sheath is slit.

By dorsiflexing the foot, the desired extent of lengthening of tendo-Achilles is achieved. Keeping the foot in zero position at ankle joint the medial and lateral cut ends of tendo-Achilles are opposed side-to-side and stitched. Paratenon is repaired as far as possible. The wound is closed and padded plaster cast is applied from mid thigh to distal end of foot by keeping the knee and ankle at 90°.

Pandey V-Y Lengthening in Continuity

It is an open procedure in which lengthening of tendinous portion of the gastroc-soleus is done at the musculotendinous junction. In this procedure a mid line incision of about 3 cm is given at the junction of lower 1/3 to upper 2/3 of the calf. The tendinous portion of the gastroc-soleus is exposed completely. While the knee is kept extended and leg elevated by about 60° from the table top, the surgeon holds the foot tightened in maximum dorsiflexed by his left hand position and by right hand only the tendinous portion of the gastroc-soleus is cut in inverted 'V' fashion. After the last few tight tendinous fibres are cut, the tendon gets lengthened and the cut ends are separated. The deeper muscular fibres also get variably stretched to provide desired lengthening of tendon. By repeated passive dorsiflexing and planterflexing of the foot the lengthening of tendon can be obviously assessed. While foot is planterflexed, the cut ends of the tendon tend to come closer and after dorsiflexing they again get separated to the lengthened extent **(Figs. 9.17A to D)**.

In this age group, almost all neglected clubfoot require some form of bony procedure over and above the soft tissue surgery (e.g. Steindler's plantar fasciotomy; tendo-Achilles lengthening; tibialis anterior (full to half) or tibialis posterior tendon transfer to the dorsolateral aspect of the foot.

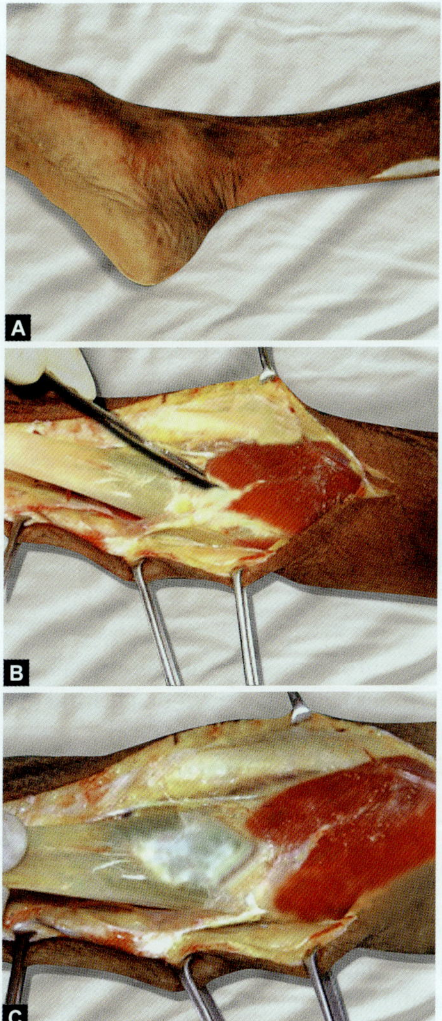

FIGS. 9.17A TO C: *Continued*

Continued

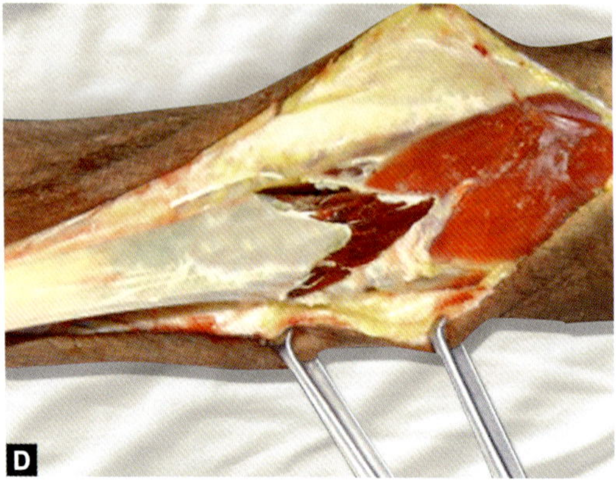

FIGS. 9.17A TO D: V-Y lengthening of tendo-Achilles as shown on fresh cadaver: (A) A mid-line incision at the lower end of gastro-soleus muscle belly over which the tendinous sheath is lying, (B) Inverted V cut is being performed, (C) Complete inverted V cut, (D) Cutting of the last tendinous fibres, the tendon gets lengthened while surgeon applies passive dorsiflexion force

In this age group the deformities are well advanced in almost all three segment of the foot, i.e. hind foot, midfoot and forefoot, besides their effect on the ankle joint. The deformities can be corrected in one stage. In such a situation the hindfoot deformity can be well corrected with the 'T' osteotomy. The midfoot deformity (mainly cavus) can be corrected by a Steindler's plantar fasciotomy with or without some bony procedures, e.g. Oblique Sliding Osteotomy-OSO (Pandey & Pandey 1984) or Japas' 'V' osteotomy (Japas 1968).

The adduction deformity, mainly confined to the forefoot, is problematic. Minor residual adduction of the forefoot can be accepted. If the adduction deformity is more prominent, it can be corrected by osteotomy through the metatarsals.

In the patients presenting with moderate cavus and clawing deformities, modified Lambrinudi (Pandey and Pandey 2002) over the original Lambrinudi (Lambrinudi 1927) type of triple arthrodesis with or without tendon transposition can be done. In the patients with severe cavus and clawing deformity, OSO of the foot can be performed as the main procedure.

CHAPTER 10

Relapsed or Recurrent Clubfoot

Despite successful treatment, relapses are common in clubfoot due to its inherent pathological tendency. Relapses are more common in stiff, severe clubfoot with small calf muscles. Most of the relapses usually occur before 5 years of age and perhaps the main reason behind this is discontinuation of night splints. Therefore, night splints are of utmost importance to prevent relapse and should be continued for at least 3–4 years of age.

RELAPSE OF CAVUS

Most of the time, this deformity is mild and can be easily corrected by manipulation and plaster cast after lifting the first metatarsal head upward. Sometimes, in more severe cases percutaneous plantar fasciotomy is performed and plaster cast is applied.

In rare cases, transfer of extensor hallucis longus tendon to the neck of the first metatarsal may be required. This will correct the plantar flexion of first metatarsal.

RELAPSE OF ADDUCTION

Most of the time recurrence of adduction of forefoot **(Fig. 10.1)** can be corrected by manipulation and two to three plaster cast applications at an interval of 2 weeks. More severe relapses require surgery either by capsulotomies at the Lisfranc's (tarsometatarsal) line or Ilizarov external fixator.

RELAPSE OF HEEL VARUS AND EQUINUS

These deformities can be corrected by manipulation and plaster cast applications to variable extent. Usually two to three plaster casts are required at an interval of 2 weeks. Foot is manipulated to keep it in extreme abduction and maximum dorsiflexion. After achieving original correction, equinus is assessed and if the dorsiflexion at ankle is less than 15°, tendo-Achilles tenotomy/lengthening should be performed. Severe relapses may need application of

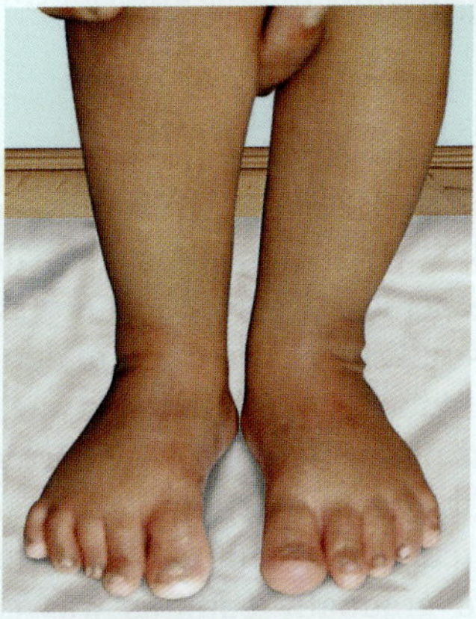

FIG. 10.1: Recurrence of adduction and cavus deformity of right foot

Ilizarov fixator to achieve correction. We encountered one case where equinus correction could not be achieved even after repeated percutaneous tendo-Achilles tenotomy, finally correction was achieved by Ilizarov fixator.

RELAPSE OF SUPINATION

Usually it can be corrected by manipulation and two to three plaster casts at an interval of 2 weeks. In those cases where navicular is not fully corrected and anteroposterior talocalcaneal angle is less than 20°, tibialis anterior has strong tendency to supinate the foot leading to greater chances of relapse. In these cases, transfer of tibialis anterior from first cuneiform and base of first metatarsal to the third cuneiform should be done in child more than 2½ years. This transfer prevents further relapse, maintains correction of heel varus, improves anteroposterior talocalcaneal angle and reduces the need for medial release operation. Joint release surgery should only be considered if relapse occurs despite tibialis anterior transfer.

Case 1

A 2-month-old baby having severe congenital clubfoot (right side) with 70° adduction, 70° equinus and 70° rotation around talus with small heel was treated by Ponseti technique. We achieved correction of cavus, adduction and heel varus fully. For correction of equinus deformity percutaneous tendo-Achilles tenotomy with plaster cast application was performed twice but correction could not be achieved. Subsequently, we applied Ilizarov fixator after performing percutaneous tendo-Achilles tenotomy for the third time and gradually equinus was corrected. After removal of frame, last plaster cast was given for 4 weeks.

After removal of plaster cast, night brace was given till the child became 4-year-old **(Figs 10.2A to C)**.

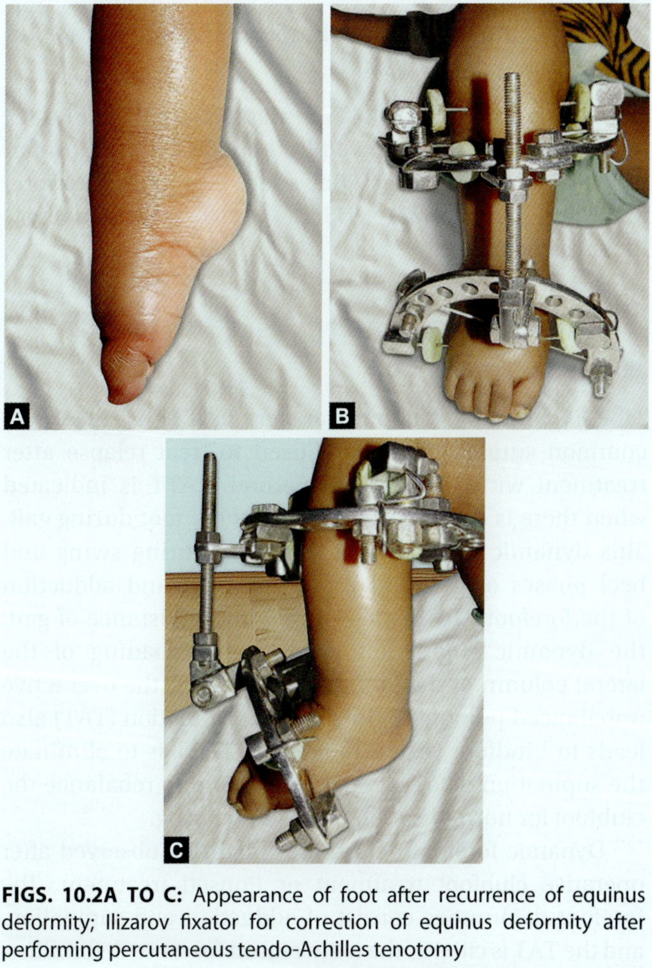

FIGS. 10.2A TO C: Appearance of foot after recurrence of equinus deformity; Ilizarov fixator for correction of equinus deformity after performing percutaneous tendo-Achilles tenotomy

TIBIALIS ANTERIOR TENDON TRANSFER FOR RELAPSED CLUBFOOT AFTER TREATMENT WITH PONSETI METHOD

Authors: Gaurav Jindal[a] MD, Bradley M Lamm[b] DPM, John E Herzenberg[c] MD, FRCSC

Corresponding Author: John E. Herzenberg, MD, FRCSC, Rubin Institute for Advanced Orthopedics, Sinai Hospital of Baltimore, 2401 West Belvedere Avenue, Baltimore, Maryland 21215-5271 USA, E-mail: jherzenberg@lifebridgehealth.org

[a]Research Fellow, [b]Head of the Section of Podiatry, [c]Head of Pediatric Orthopedics

Introduction

Tibialis anterior tendon transfer (TATT) is the most common surgical procedure used to treat relapse after treatment with the Ponseti method. TATT is indicated when there is dynamic supination of the foot during gait. This dynamic supination is observed during swing and heel phases of gait and produces varus and adduction of the forefoot. During heel strike and midstance of gait, the dynamic supination produces overloading of the lateral column of the foot. In severe cases, the overactive unbalanced pull of the tibialis anterior tendon (TAT) also leads to hindfoot varus. The aim of TATT is to eliminate the supination deformity of the foot and to rebalance the clubfoot for normalisation of weight bearing.

Dynamic forefoot deformities might be observed after operative clubfoot treatment or Ponseti treatment. The forefoot deformities consist of adduction and supination, and the TAT is cited as the main reason for these deformities.

A dynamic deformity should be differentiated from a rigid deformity, which often results from bony deformity or joint contracture. A dynamic deformity is the result of weak peroneal muscles and an imbalance of muscle function from an unopposed TAT. Feldbrin et al., conducted electrophysiological studies on 52 pediatric patients with idiopathic clubfoot and concluded that 27% of the patients experienced isolated peroneal nerve dysfunction.

Dynamic forefoot supination can be explained biomechanically. The TAT straddles the longitudinal axis of the subtalar joint, thereby producing a dorsiflexion moment on the ankle **(Fig. 10.3)**. When the subtalar joint is pronated or supinated, the pull of the TAT is shifted lateral or medial to this axis, respectively. Because of the weak

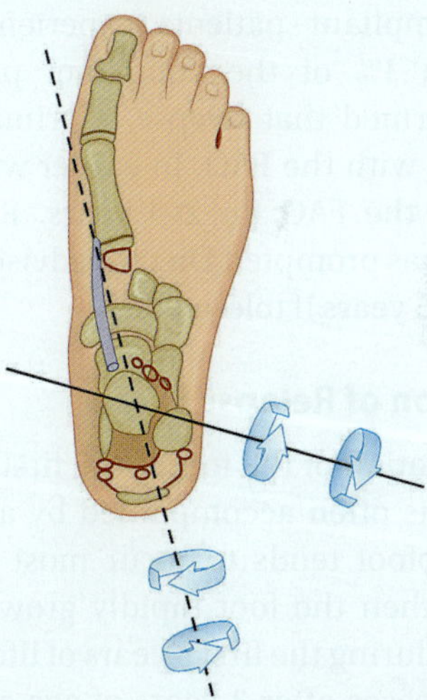

FIG. 10.3: Position of TAT just medial to subtalar axis makes it a strong supinator in clubfoot that has already a supinated subtalar joint

lateral muscle group, the supination of the clubfoot shifts the TAT medial to the subtalar joint longitudinal axis. This shift in the TAT produces more supination.

Pathogenesis of Relapse

Relapse seems to be the consequence of muscular imbalance. It has also been observed that relapse is most common in severe cases of clubfoot or when the patient has a small calf size. Relapses typically occur in toddlers, but they can occur in children as old as 6–8 years.

After a foot has been successfully corrected with the Ponseti method, it is critical to maintain the correction with the use of a foot abduction orthosis (FAO) for 4 years. Morcuende et al studied patients who were treated with the Ponseti method from 1991 to 2001 and found that 89% of noncompliant patients experienced a relapse compared with 1% of the compliant patients. Dobbs et al also confirmed that relapse is primarily related to noncompliance with the FAO. In earlier writings, Ponseti advised use of the FAO for 2–4 years. Recent research about relapses has prompted Dietz to advise use of the FAO until the age of 5 years if tolerated.

Presentation of Relapse

Dynamic supination of the foot is the first clinical sign of relapse, and it is often accompanied by a slight equinus deformity. Clubfoot tends to recur most frequently and most quickly when the foot rapidly grows. Relapses are most common during the first 3 years of life. The incidence of relapse decreases after 3 years of age and is rare after 6 years of age. The parents often report that it is difficult to apply the FAO to a relapsed clubfoot.

Observe the child as he or she walks. As the child walks towards you, look for elevation of the medial column and as the child walks away from you, look for heel varus. The dynamic deformity can also be demonstrated in a seated child by observing unbalanced first ray elevation when the patient attempts to dorsiflex the foot voluntarily. In addition, the skin on the plantar aspect of the foot should be observed carefully. A lack of callus beneath the great toe joint is a sign of supination. We ask the child to walk barefoot in our clinic and then examine the plantar aspect of the foot to see if dust has accumulated in the weight bearing regions of the foot. If the child is walking with dynamic supination, no dust will be observed beneath the great toe. Alternatively, it is possible to determine the presence of dynamic supination with a pedobarographic study.

Treatment of Relapse

The initial treatment for relapsed clubfoot in a patient younger than 2.5 years is to immediately recast using Ponseti method. Long leg casts are changed every 1 to 2 weeks. If the Achilles tendon remains tight after casting, it might require repeat tenotomy or open tendo-Achilles lengthening. In a patient older than 2.5 years, relapse can be treated with TATT to the third cuneiform because the third cuneiform starts to ossify at this age. In addition, an Achilles tendon lengthening or gastrocnemius-soleus recession can be performed concurrently for treatment of equinus. TATT to the third cuneiform underneath the extensor retinaculum corrects and stabilises the foot by restoring normal eversion function. Full transfer of the tendon should be performed just lateral to midline to allow dorsiflexion without excessive abduction. This transfer might produce loss of dorsiflexion strength by one grade, which might become functionally important if residual equinus is present. Thus, assessment of ankle joint contracture and the posterior muscle group is necessary. If tight, these structures are released to prevent a more significant equinus.

Idiopathic clubfoot can relapse regardless of the treatment and the adequacy of the correction achieved. A high incidence of relapse has been reported, even in feet that achieved a full correction during the first month of life. Approximately 10–20% of clubfeet require TATT even after being treated with the Ponseti method. If left untreated, the dynamic deformity tends to become stiff.

Fixed deformity of the foot must be corrected before performing TATT. This correction is typically achieved with two or three casts before performing the transfer. If the foot has undergone open posteromedial release, casting might or might not correct the deformity of the foot. If correction is not achieved, then surgical procedures that address bony deformities might be required before performing TATT.

History of Tibialis Anterior Tendon Transfer

In 1940, Garceau first described performing TATT to treat recurrent idiopathic clubfoot. Three incisions were made: One over the tibialis anterior tendon close to its distal insertion, a second incision at the level of the musculotendinous junction, and a third incision over the junction of the fifth metatarsal with the cuboid. The tendon was detached from its original insertion and pulled out through the second incision. It was then moved to the lateral side of the foot and anchored to the base of the fifth metatarsal or to the cuboid, possibly beneath the extensor retinaculum at the ankle, although this was not absolutely necessary.

Garceau reported short- and long-term results in two additional studies and concluded that TATT to the lateral aspect of the foot was a useful procedure to correct relapsing deformities. He reported that 77% of patients achieved good or excellent results in forefoot adduction correction and 93% in inversion deformity correction. Since then, TATT has been widely used for the management of residual clubfoot deformity.

Ponseti and Smoley in 1963 modified Garceau's surgical technique by always performing the transfer to the third cuneiform and without rerouting the tendon under the lateral part of the extensor retinaculum. In 1974, Hoffer et al first described split TATT to treat children with cerebral palsy who experienced spastic varus hindfoot deformity. Laaveg and Ponseti in 1980 reported good results in a long-term follow-up study of relapsing clubfeet treated with full TATT. Cooper and Dietz in 1995 confirmed these results in the same series of patients who were reviewed 30 years after treatment. Ricciardi–Pollini et al in 1984 and Ippolito et al in 1985 studied the same series of patients and stated that TATT to the third cuneiform is the most effective procedure to prevent and correct relapses for cases of idiopathic clubfoot. Ezra et al in 2000 reported a series of 27 feet treated with TATT for dynamic recurrence of clubfoot deformity and followed the cases for 2 to 14 years after surgery. At follow-up, none of the patients experienced dynamic supination deformity during gait. Kuo et al in 2001 reported clinical and radiographic improvement in both forefoot adduction and supination in 71 cases of residual dynamic clubfoot deformity treated with either full or split TATT. They also noted an increase of the eversion strength of the TAT. Farsetti et al evaluated 25 patients with 35 relapsing clubfeet. The patients were treated with TATT to the third cuneiform by using the Ponseti and Smoley technique. Farsetti et al observed better outcomes at maturity when the relapsing deformity was passively correctable at the time of surgery.

Timing of Surgical Intervention

TATT should be performed when the foot starts to relapse, which prevents worsening of the relapsed deformity and stiffness of the foot. However, the procedure cannot be performed until an ossified third cuneiform is present radiographically (typically present in children older than 2.5 years). TATT is advisable when the ossific nucleus of third cuneiform is sufficiently large enough to accommodate the bony tunnel, which avoids damaging the ossific nucleus and ensures good tendon to bone healing.

Types of Tibialis Anterior Tendon Transfer

In Garceau's original article, he transferred the tendon onto the fifth metatarsal bone unless the tendon was too short; in such cases, he transferred it onto the cuboid bone. Laaveg and Ponseti, in their long-term results of treatment of idiopathic clubfoot, reported full transfer of the tibialis anterior tendon to the lateral cuneiform to prevent recurrence. Ponseti thought that TATT to the fifth metatarsal or cuboid might result in excessive foot eversion. Hoffer et al performed split tibialis anterior tendon transfer onto the cuboid bone. Kuo et al preferred transfer to the lateral cuneiform for the full tendon transfer and to the cuboid bone for the split-tendon transfer.

Hui et al in their biomechanical study of 10 normal anatomic specimens, concluded that for the full transfer, the ideal site of insertion was along the third metatarsal axis as described by Ponseti. They found that this location allowed for the greatest amount of dorsiflexion and eversion. Ponseti advocates full transfer of the tibialis anterior tendon to the third cuneiform and thinks that splitting the tendon causes dorsiflexion but does not correct forefoot supination.

Preoperative Treatment

If the foot is completely supple and correctable, the surgeon can perform TATT without initial casting or surgical treatment. Initially, most relapsed clubfeet are not passively correctable. If the deformity has a fixed or resistant component, preoperative casting is indicated to correct the deformity. Ponseti long leg casts are usually applied biweekly so that passive correction can be achieved before performing TATT. It can be challenging to apply a cast to an older child who is both strong and uncooperative. If indicated, tendo-Achillis lengthening or gastrocnemius-soleus recession can be performed to allow maximum dorsiflexion of the ankle. The tendo-Achillis lengthening or gastrocnemius-soleus recession can be performed before TATT at the same surgical setting.

Surgical Technique

Child is placed in supine position on a radiolucent table under general anaesthesia. A tourniquet is inflated after exsanguinating the limb with an Esmarch bandage. A 3 cm longitudinal incision is made along the course of tibialis anterior tendon from the inferior margin of the extensor retinaculum to its distal insertion **(Fig. 10.4A)**.

The tendon is detached from its insertion into the first cuneiform and first metatarsal to ensure adequate length. Care should be taken not to open the cuneiform first metatarsal joint and also not to damage the physis at the base of the first metatarsal. The distal end of the detached tendon is held by a hemostat or a small Kocher clamp and lifted from its sheath up to its compartment under the superior extensor retinaculum. Care is taken to leave the extensor retinaculum intact. An anchoring suture is placed in the distal 2.5 cm of the TATT in a whip-stitch fashion **(Figs 10.4B and C)**. The TATT is measured for the maximum width with a tendon sizer.

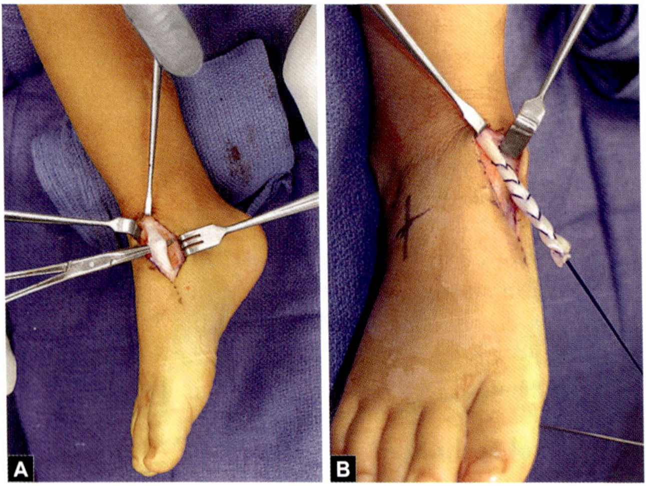

FIGS 10.4A AND B: Operative technique for TATT. (A) Tibialis anterior tendon is identified and dissected through a 3 cm longitudinal incision and then released at its insertion. (B) Tibialis anterior tendon is anchored with No. 1 polydioxanone suture (PDS) by using a whip stitch suture technique

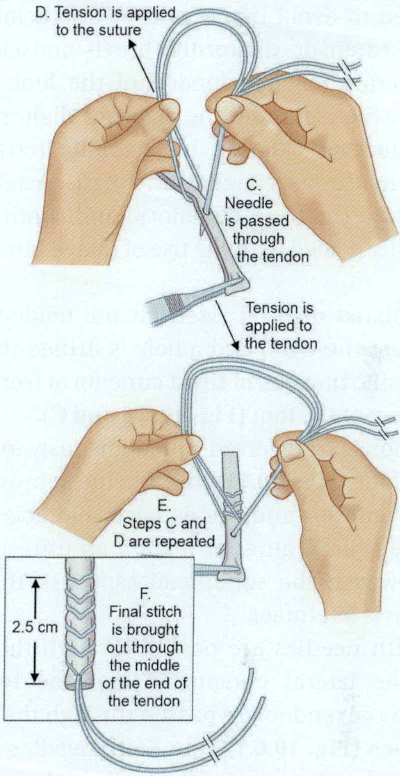

FIG. 10.4C: Whip stitch suture technique for securing the tibialis anterior tendon

The third cuneiform is then identified clinically by palpating the third metatarsal base and feeling for the joint between the third metatarsal and the third cuneiform. Image intensification is also used to confirm the location of the third cuneiform before making the second incision. A second 2.5 cm longitudinal incision is made at this level.

Care is taken to avoid injury to the superficial peroneal nerve. The extensor digitorum brevis muscle belly is elevated laterally off the dorsum of the foot. The third cuneiform, which is under the extensor digitorum brevis muscle, is further exposed by medially retracting the tendons of the extensor digitorum longus. A 1.5-mm wire is inserted into the third cuneiform and confirmed to be concentrically placed with the use of image intensification **(Fig. 10.5A)**.

A cannulated drill bit sized for the tendon diameter is passed over the wire, and a hole is drilled through the centre of ossific nucleus of third cuneiform from dorsal to plantar aspect of the foot **(Figs 10.5B and C)**.

The tendon is transferred subcutaneously to the lateral side of the foot **(Figs 10.5D and E)**. The septum between the tibialis anterior and the extensor hallucis is divided to allow the tibialis anterior tendon an unrestricted line of pull. However, the superficial aspect of the extensor retinaculum is left intact.

Two Keith needles are passed through the drill hole made in the lateral cuneiform, and the two sutures anchored to the tendon are passed through the eyes of the Keith needles **(Fig. 10.6A)**. The Keith needles are passed through the plantar aspect of the foot and through a sterile foam pad and suture button **(Fig. 10.6B)**. Readily available sterile disposable scrub brushes without soap are used to fashion the foam pad of 2.5 cm cube size to protect the plantar skin from the hard plastic button. The two needles are then removed. Next, the tendon is inset. This is the most critical part of the procedure. We recommend insetting the tendon with the foot held in maximum dorsiflexion and eversion. After the tendon has been inset, care should be taken to prevent inadvertent plantar flexion of the

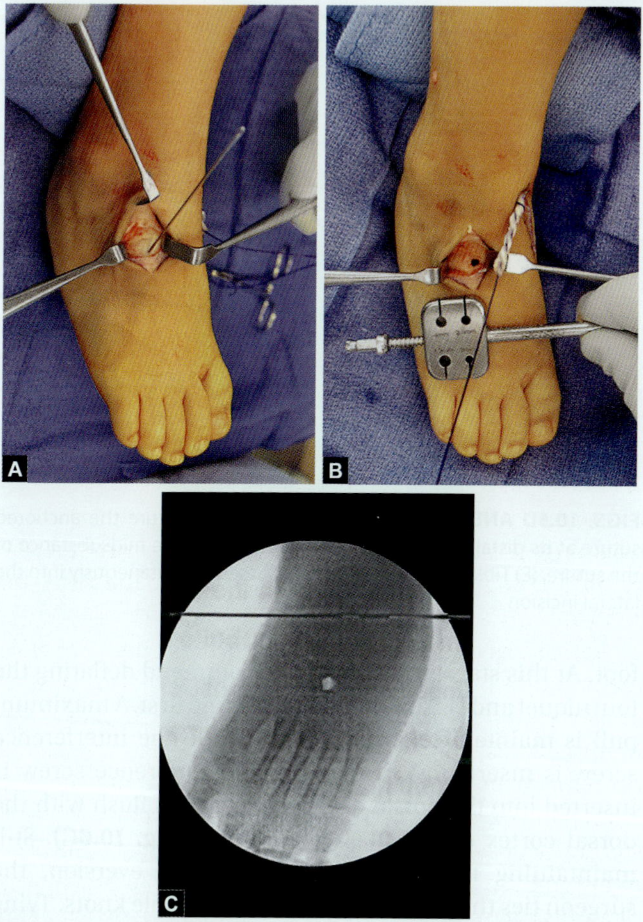

FIGS. 10.5A TO C: (A) Second longitudinal incision is made over the lateral cuneiform. After dissection, a guide pin is inserted in the centre of ossific nucleus of lateral cuneiform under fluoroscopic guidance. (B) Lateral cuneiform has been drilled with an appropriate sized cannulated drill bit. Note the tendon sizer. (C) Intraoperative view using an image intensifier shows a drill hole centered on the lateral cuneiform

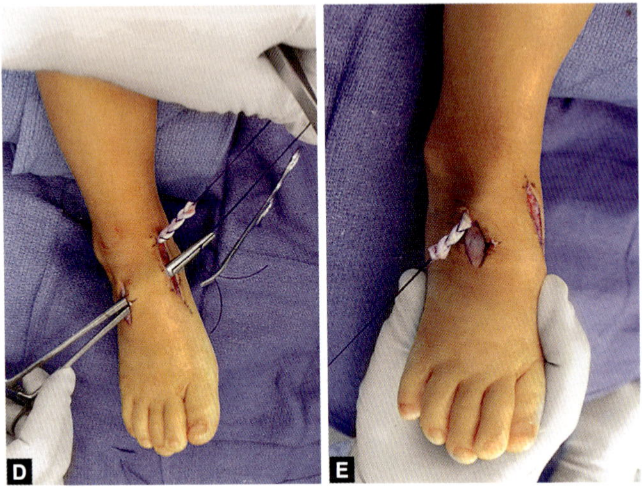

FIGS. 10.5D AND E: (D) Hemostat is used to capture the anchored suture at its distal-most end, so as not to weaken the midsubstance of the suture. (E) Tibialis anterior tendon is passed subcutaneously into the lateral incision

foot. At this stage, therefore, we recommend deflating the tourniquet and closing the medial wound first. A maximum pull is maintained on the suture while the interference screw is inserted. A bioabsorbable interference screw is inserted into the dorsal drill hole until it is flush with the dorsal cortex of the lateral cuneiform **(Fig. 10.6C)**. Still maintaining maximum dorsiflexion and eversion, the surgeon ties the plantar sutures with multiple knots. Tying the knots too tightly can lead to pressure necrosis of the skin under the button. By having an interference screw holding the tendon, the need to overtighten the suture for fixation is decreased.

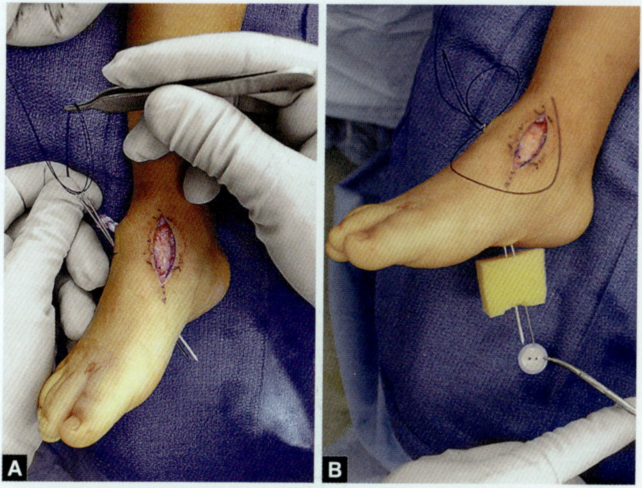

FIGS. 10.6A AND B: (A) Two Keith needles are passed through the drill hole from dorsal to plantar side. The sutures anchored to the tibialis anterior tendon are then passed through the eyes of the Keith needles. (B) Tibialis anterior tendon is pulled into the drill hole. The two suture ends are then passed through the sole of the foot and through a foam pad and button. The sutures are tied only after the placement of the screw

After the suture has been inserted and tightened, the tibialis anterior tendon typically measures approximately 4.5 mm in diameter. The hole is drilled with a 4.5 or 4.8 mm cannulated drill bit. A Bio-Tenodesis absorbable interference screw (Arthrex Inc., Florida, USA) with a diameter of 4.75 mm and a length of 15 mm is used. We prefer to use strong No. 1 slowly absorbable monofilament suture material [e.g. monocryl or polydioxanone suture (PDS) (Ethicon Inc., Johnson and Johnson, Somerville, New Jersey, USA)]. Our rationale for this choice is that when

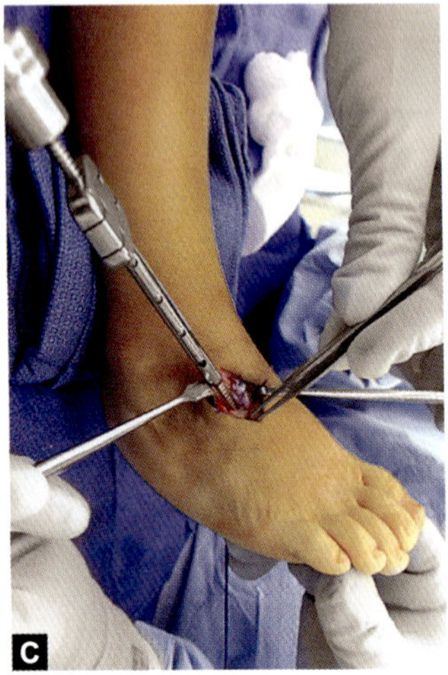

FIG. 10.6C: A bio-absorbable screw is inserted while maintaining maximal traction on the suture and while maximally dorsiflexing and everting the foot

the suture is removed at 6 weeks, any residual portion that breaks off and resists removal will be absorbed, making it less likely to be a nidus of infection.

Two methods of complementary fixation (i.e. interference screw and suture tied over a button) are used to secure the tendon and to increase the strength of the fixation. We call this technique "belt and suspenders". Two methods of tendon fixation lessen the risk of tendon pull out, loosening, or failure.

After surgery, a long leg Ponseti cast is applied with the foot in neutral position and the knee at 90° of flexion. The anaesthetist is asked to keep the child deeply asleep until the cast dries. The patient should not bear any weight on the operated foot for 6 weeks. The cast, the suture, and the button are removed at 6 weeks, and the child is allowed weight bearing as tolerated while wearing a regular shoe. Physiotherapy is sometimes needed to obtain maximal early rehabilitation.

Discussion

1. Transfer of the TATT out of its compartment, superficial to the extensor retinaculum, will create bowstring of the tendon under the skin in front of the ankle. This bowstring phenomenon might decrease the motor strength of the TATT and often causes tendon irritation. We avoid the tendon bowstring phenomenon by keeping the tendon beneath the extensor retinaculum.
2. We use the whip stitch suture technique. We avoid a Bunnell crisscross suture because when the tendon is prepared with this technique and pulled, it produces a concertina effect on the tendon, thereby decreasing its effective length and increasing the diameter. The whip stitch suture technique is less traumatic to the tendon and is easy to perform.
3. The risk of tendon pull out is minimised by the "belt and suspenders" technique of double fixation described above. The interference screw and the suture tied over a button provide combined stability to resist tendon pull out. If the above mentioned technique is used, pressure necrosis on the plantar skin below the button is rarely observed.

Conclusion

Clubfoot relapses will occur and can be more effectively and easily treated if recognised promptly. The relapsed clubfoot must be well corrected by using Ponseti manipulations and by applying plaster casts before performing tendon transfer. TATT provides balanced muscular control with dorsiflexion. TATT does not change the axial direction of the muscle function and does not change the phasic pattern of the tibialis anterior tendon during walking. After tendon transfer, bracing with the FAO is no longer required because the correction is maintained by the eversion force vector of the transferred tendon. TATT also prevents further relapses. Because the tibialis anterior tendon is joint sparing, the foot retains its suppleness and maximal strength. In long-term follow-up studies of patients treated with TATT, the procedure did not compromise the outcome with respect to level of pain and functional limitations.

CHAPTER 11

Secondary Clubfoot and Other Conditions

INTRODUCTION

Syndromic clubfoot is secondary to a condition that affects our muscles or skeleton, such as arthrogryposis, constriction band syndrome, tibial hemimelia, and diastrophic dwarfism.

Conditions associated with secondary or syndromic clubfoot are as follows:

- Neurogenic causes (spina bifida, meningomyelocele, and diastematomyelia)
- Myogenic causes
- Tibia hemimelia
- Amniotic band syndrome (Streeter's dysplasia)
- Pierre Robin syndrome
- Opitz syndrome
- Larsen syndrome
- Prune–Belly syndrome
- Anterior tibia artery hypoplasia/absent

Treatment in these types of feet also starts with standard Ponseti method.

But, some types of these feet are more resistant to conservative treatment, sometimes they need soft-tissue procedures or bony procedures or Ilizarov technique. They need long term of course, more casts than normal, long duration of brace time. Results are also not expected as in idiopathic clubfoot. Because in these feet, pathoanatomy is different than in idiopathic clubfoot. Muscles are short in size and ligaments and capsules are more fibrotic in nature.

ARTHROGRYPOSIS MULTIPLEX CONGENITA (FIG. 11.1)

Arthrogryposis multiplex congenita (AMC) pathophysiologically begins with failure of fetal movement usually caused by failure of development of anterior horn cells at spinal level. Anterior horn cells are diminished in number, but they remain normal in appearance. It is seen that ventral roots are decreased in number while dorsal roots are normal. Joints and articular cartilages are well formed but capsules are thickened and fibrotic, joint creases are

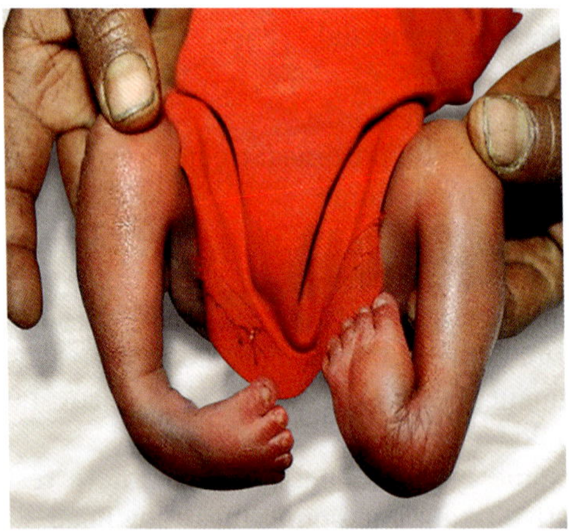

FIG. 11.1: Arthrogryposis multiplex congenita (AMC) with bilateral clubfoot

absent, bursae are underdeveloped, tendons are often fibrosed to their sheaths, muscles are thinned, atrophic, and at times infiltrated with fat. Affected muscles are firm, pale, fibrous and show fatty degeneration.

Most common foot deformity associated with AMC is equinovarus (clubfoot), which is more rigid than idiopathic variety. Other foot deformities are vertical talus, equinovalgus and cavus. In knee, flexion contracture is more frequent, but extension contracture, hyperextension, varus, and valgus deformities are also common.

Management

A well-planned conservative and surgical management should be adopted for treating this syndrome. Ideally, the treatment should be completed by the age of 6–7 years.

Deformities of foot (clubfoot) should be treated by manipulation followed by plaster cast application by Ponseti technique. Some of the rigid clubfoot not corrected by plaster casts may need early surgical release or correction by Ilizarov ring fixator. Associated knee flexion contracture is treated by stretching exercises, splints, and supracondylar femoral osteotomy fixed with Ilizarov fixator in severe cases.

Case 1

A 5-month-old female child having arthrogryposis multiplex congenita with clubfoot deformity (left side) (resistant clubfoot) was brought to OPD. She was treated by Ponseti technique by manipulation and plaster cast application followed by percutaneous tendo-Achilles tenotomy. Her clubfoot deformity was corrected in normal course of time. She was put in Steenbeck abduction brace till 2 years of age. She was operated for flexion deformity of knee by supracondylar femoral osteotomy fixed with Ilizarov ring fixator. During the treatment of flexion deformity of knee, due to discontinuation of brace she developed recurrence of cavus and adduction which were corrected by serial plaster casts **(Figs. 11.2A to Q)**.

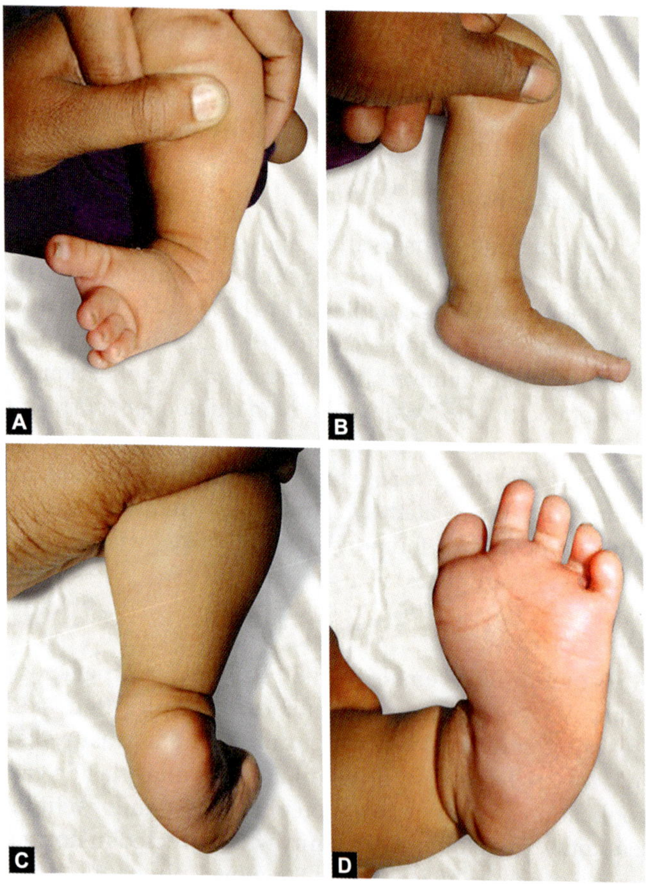

FIGS. 11.2A TO D: Pretreatment photographs

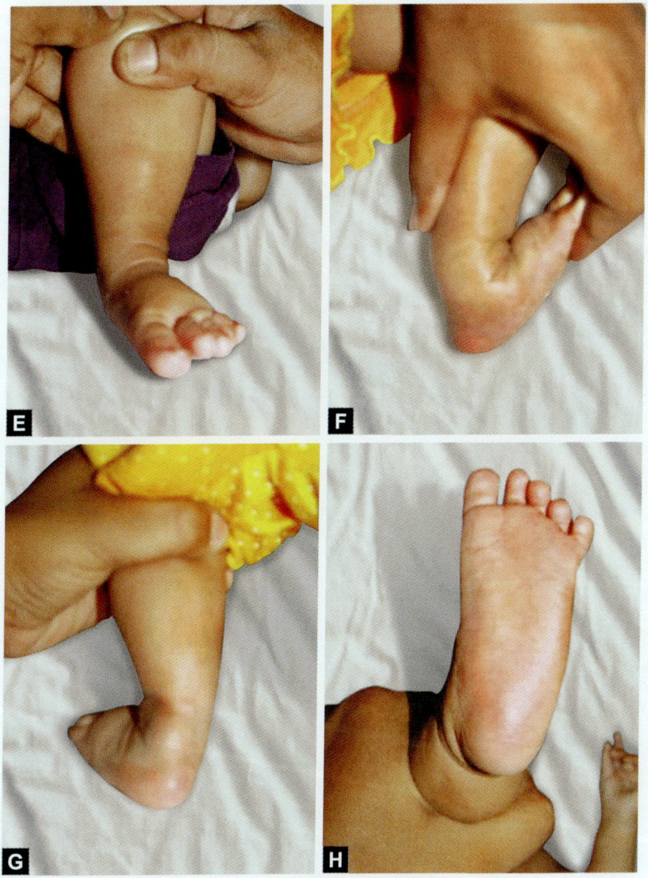

FIGS. 11.2E TO H: After Ponseti cast

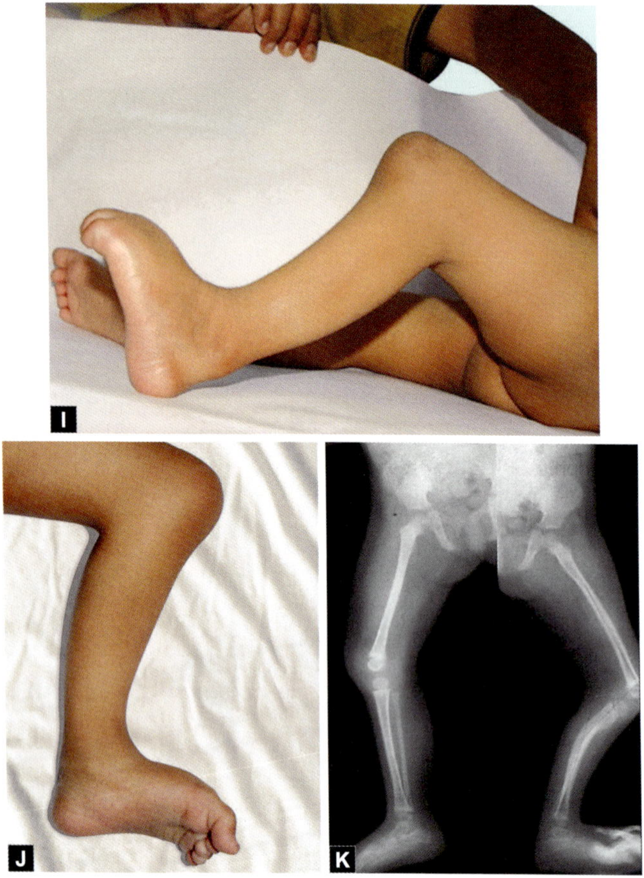

FIGS. 11.2I TO K: Flexion deformity due to arthrogryposis multiplex congenita (AMC)

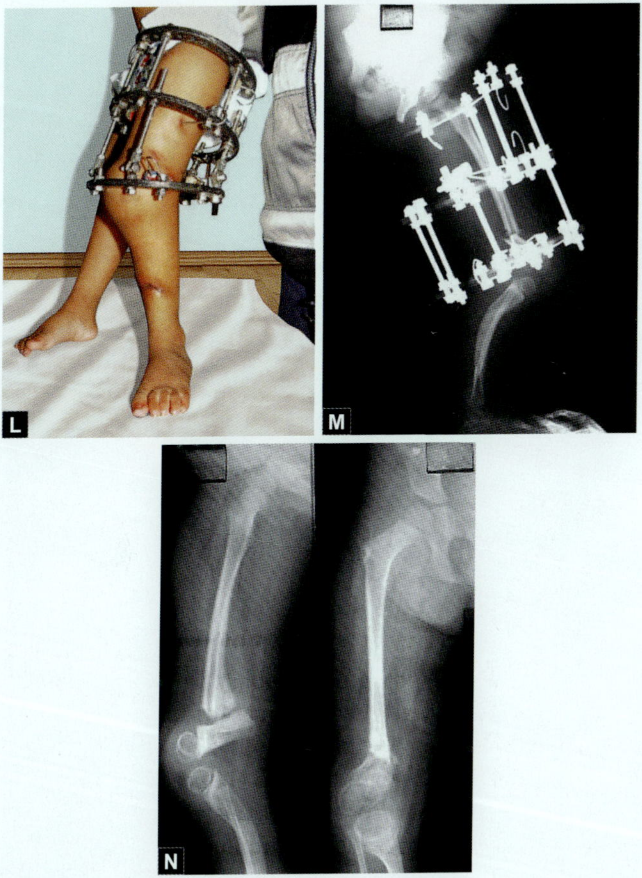

FIGS. 11.2L TO N: Supracondylar osteotomy for correction of flexion deformity

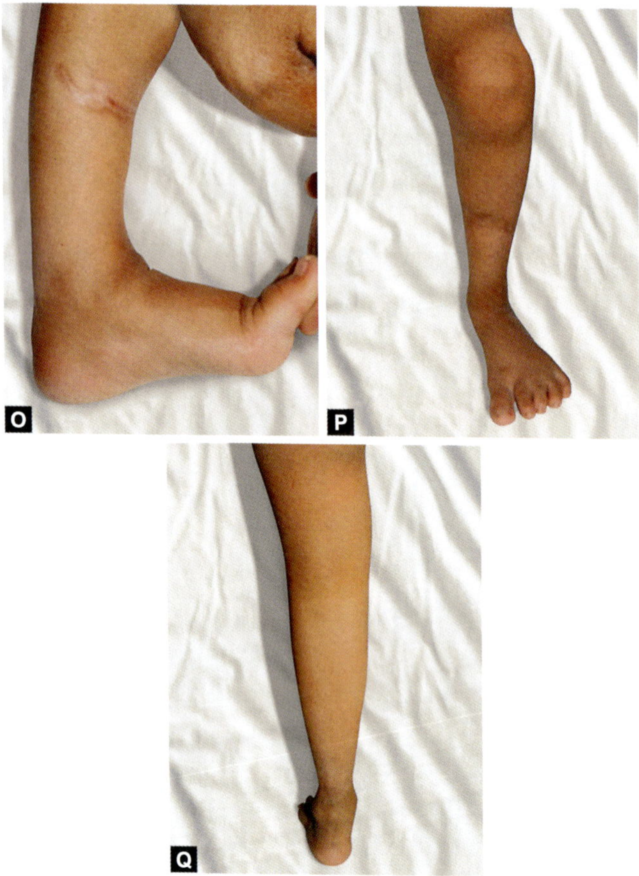

FIGS. 11.2O TO Q: Final photographs after complete treatment

SPINA BIFIDA (FIGS. 3A TO H)

In patients with spina bifida, clubfoot is the most common foot deformity and has been reported to occur in 30–50% of patients. Many factors may contribute to the development of clubfoot in patients with spina bifida, including spasticity, intrauterine positioning, contractures, and muscle imbalance. For instance, in a patient with low-lumbar level of involvement, clubfoot may develop due to either retained activity or contracture of the tibialis muscles in combination with the functional absence of the peroneal muscles. Additionally, the incidence of clubfoot varies with the neurologic level of involvement of the patient. Clubfoot occurs in approximately 90% of patients with thoracic or lumbar levels of involvement and 50% of patients with sacral level involvement. Consideration for open rather than a percutaneous approach is recommended for the tendo-Achilles to allow for the excision of at least 1 cm of tendon to prevent the recurrence of equinus.

Role of Ilizarov

Case 1

Ilizarov fixator was applied in leg and foot. Gradually, deformity was corrected by Ponseti principles. First forefoot and midfoot which was in pronation was supinated by rotation. When the pronation was corrected and configuration was changed, then the forefoot and midfoot was abducted by gradual differential distraction to achieve 30–40° of abduction. As soon as abduction achieved, varus heel was corrected. V-Y plasty of gastrosoleus was done. Followed by ankle arthrodesis with retrograde nailing was done. There was a contracture of big toe which was treated with arthrodesis of metatarsophalangeal and interphalangeal joint and fixed with K wire.

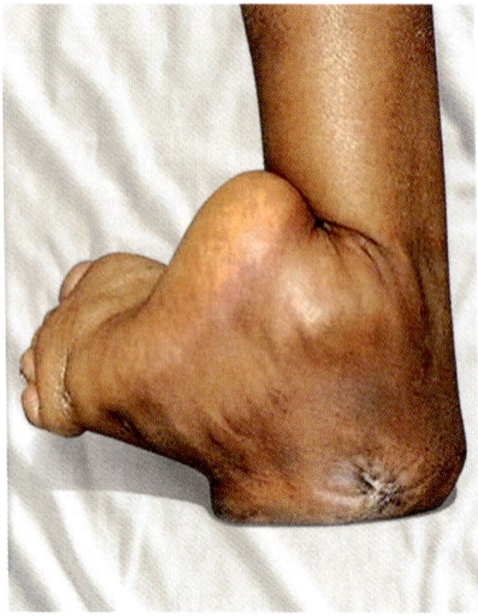

FIG. 11.3A: Neurogenic neglected clubfoot

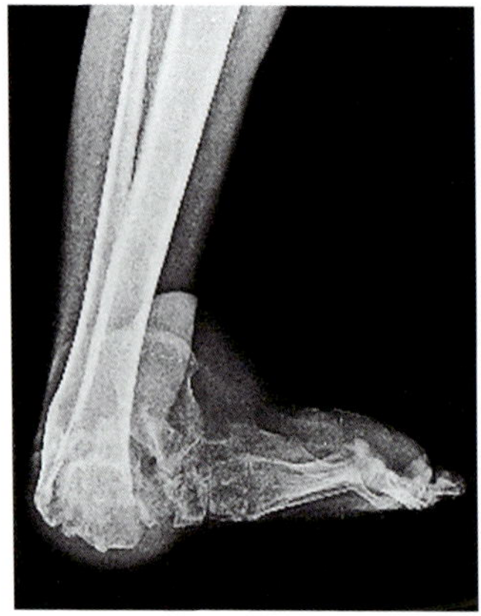

FIG. 11.3B: Radiograph neglected clubfoot

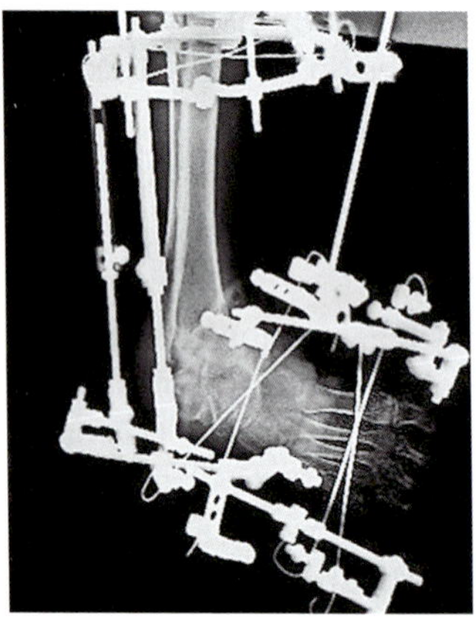

FIG. 11.3C: Radiograph with ilizarov

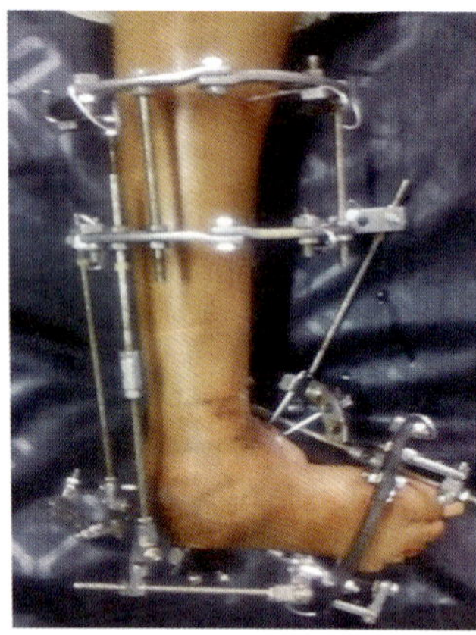

FIG. 11.3D: Clinical photograph with ilizarov

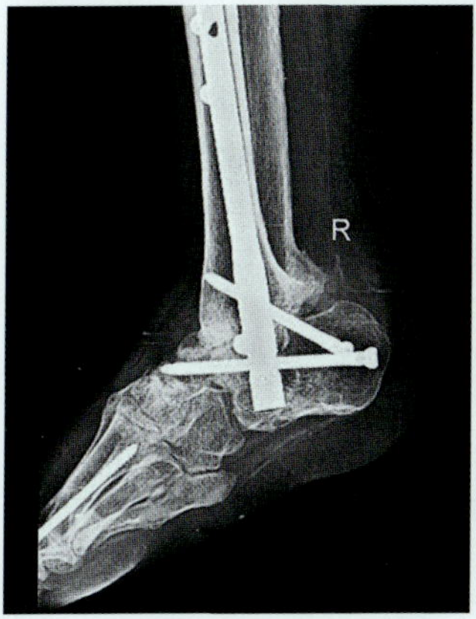

FIG. 11.3E: Final X-ray showing ankle arthrodesis lateral view

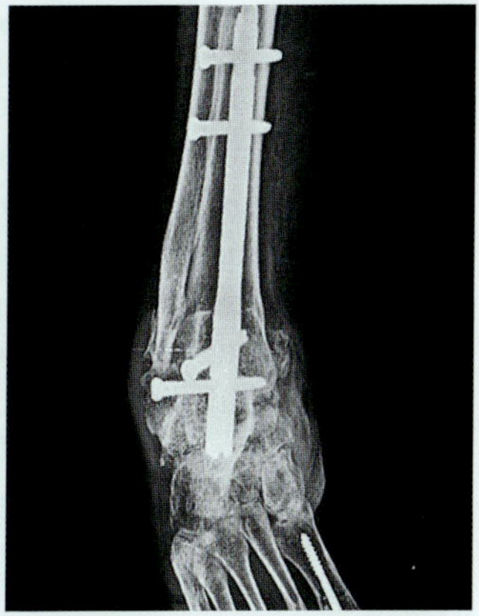

FIG. 11.3F: Final X-ray showing ankle arthrodesis anteroposterior (AP) view

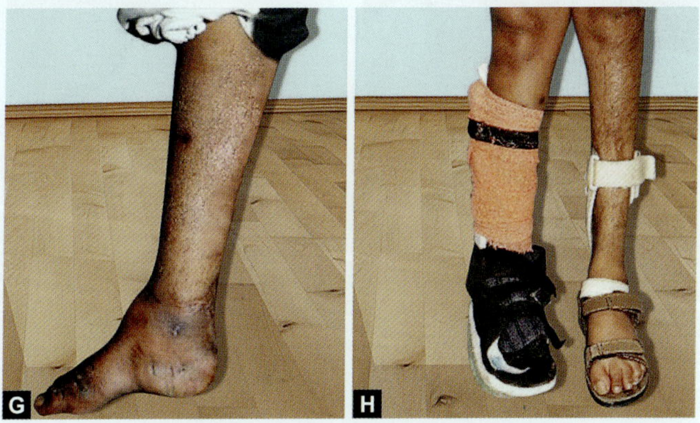

FIGS. 11.3G AND H: Final photographs

AMNIOTIC BAND SYNDROME (FIGS. 4A TO C)

The cause of this syndrome is not fully clear, children with this condition are born with tight skin and soft-tissue bands around their limbs which lead to constricting blood and lymph flow causing swelling. In this syndrome, upper limbs are more involved than lower limbs. The feet responded favorably to casting although equinus correction required more extensive surgical interventions. The preexisting edema in distal limb often precluded a snuggly fitting cast increasing the cast numbers. Careful monitoring of vascularity is essential. Simultaneous procedures of release of constriction bands, correction of hand anomalies, and equinus can be combined to give advantage to the patient.

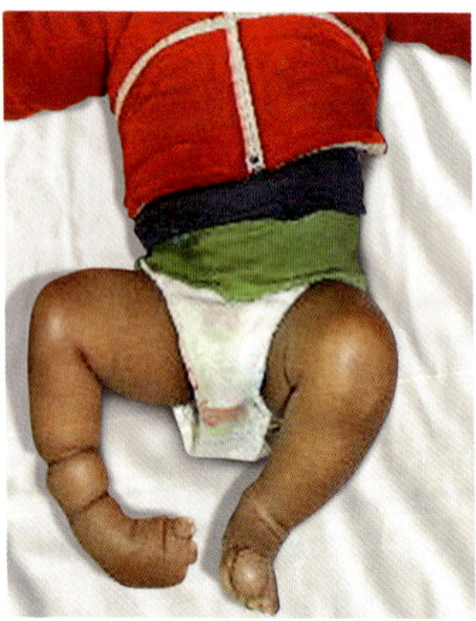

FIG. 11.4A: Clinical photo with amniotic band syndrome

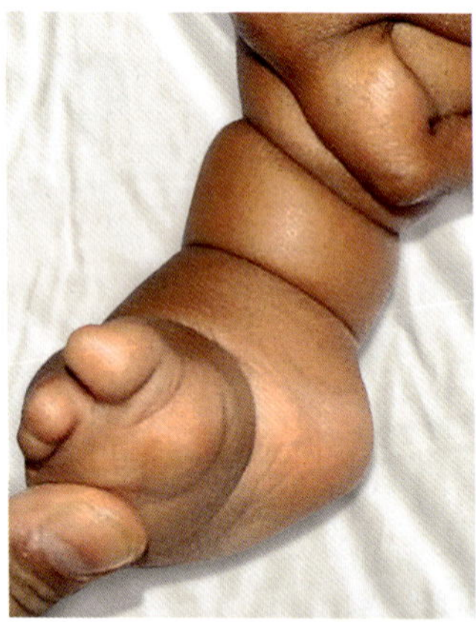

FIG. 11.4B: Clinical photo with amniotic band syndrome: Anterior view

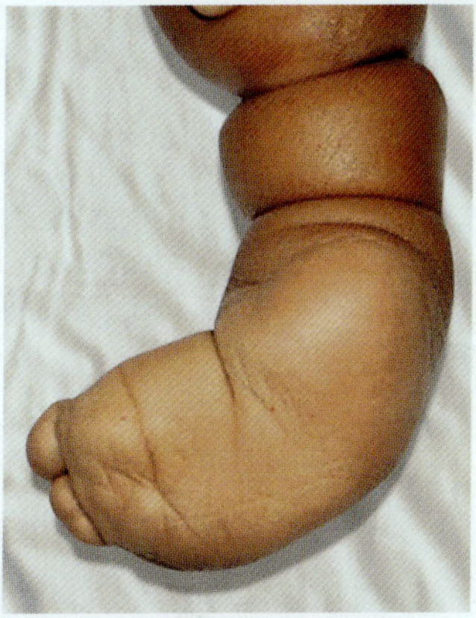

FIG. 11.4C: Clinical photo with amniotic band syndrome: Posterior view

TIBIAL HEMIMELIA (FIG. 5)

It is a condition where development and formation of tibia affected from complete agenesis to mild agenesis. This condition is associated with short tibia, bowing of leg, femur, and foot abnormalities also. So, basically in sometimes bowing of tibia with shortening looks like clubfoot which is ruled out by clinical examination and X-rays. But, patients who are having clubfoot are treated with standard Ponseti method. Some cases are resistant to conservative treatment because of association with tarsal coalition, and tight soft-tissue structures conditions. Requires extensive soft-tissue release, bony procedures, or Ilizarov.

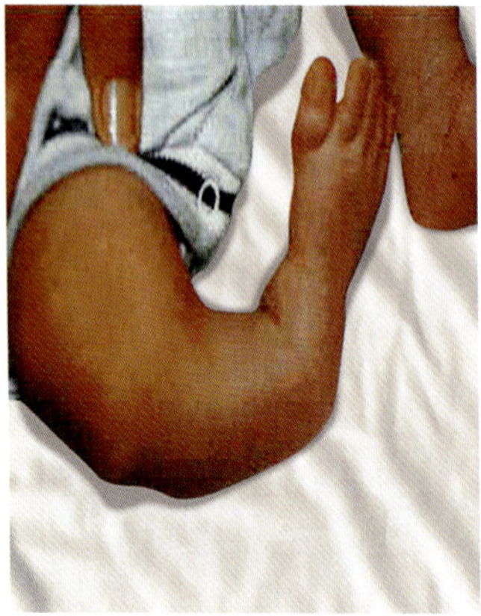

FIG. 11.5: Showing clubfoot with tibia agenesis

CHAPTER 12

Errors and Complications

INTRODUCTION

Errors and complications are part and parcel of any skill, but they can be avoided by understanding the pathological anatomy and manipulation with the help of model, because a faulty treatment not only fails but also makes clubfoot stiffer which becomes very difficult to treat.

MOST FREQUENT ERRORS DURING MANIPULATION AND CAST APPLICATION

1. *Pronating the forefoot rather supinating and abducting it*: Forefoot pronation increases cavus and makes this deformity more rigid as plantar fascia thickens and tightens. Pronation does not help to abduct the adducted and inverted calcaneus, which remains locked under the talus. It also produces a new deformity of eversion through the midfoot and forefoot, leading to a bean-shaped foot **(Fig. 12.1)**.
2. *External rotation (abduction) of foot to correct adduction while calcaneus remains in varus*: This happens when we manipulate (abduct) the foot by holding ankle

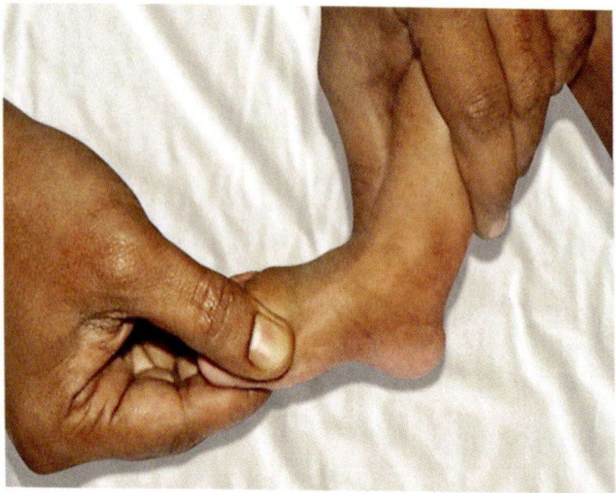

FIG. 12.1: Pronating forefoot instead of supination

instead of giving counterpressure at lateral head of talus. This causes a posterior displacement of the lateral malleolus by externally rotating the talus in the ankle mortise. Avoid this problem by abducting the foot in slight supination to stretch the medial tarsal ligaments with counterpressure applied on the lateral aspect of the head of the talus. This allows the calcaneus to abduct under the talus with correction of the heel varus **(Fig. 12.2)**.

3. *Abducting the foot at midtarsal joints with the thumb pressing on the lateral side of the foot near the calcaneo-cuboid joint (Ponseti suggested it to be the Kite's error)*: Kite believed that the heel varus would correct simply by everting the calcaneum. He did not realise that the calcaneum can evert only when it is abducted under the talus.

   Abducting the foot at the midtarsal joints with the thumb pressing on the lateral side of the foot near

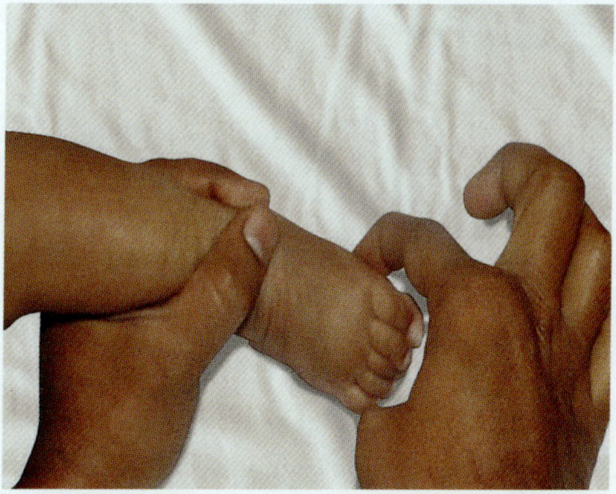

FIG. 12.2: Malpractice by manipulating foot with holding at ankle joint

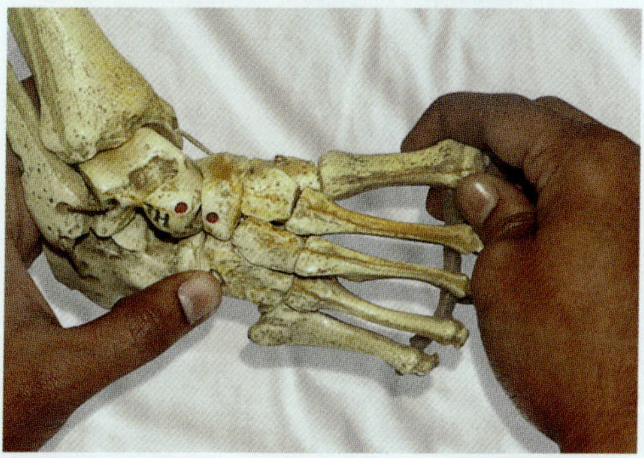

FIG. 12.3A: Bone model showing applying pressure at calcaneo-cuboid joint

the calcaneocuboid joint blocks abduction of the calcaneum and interferes with correction of the heel varus **(Figs. 12.3A and B)**.

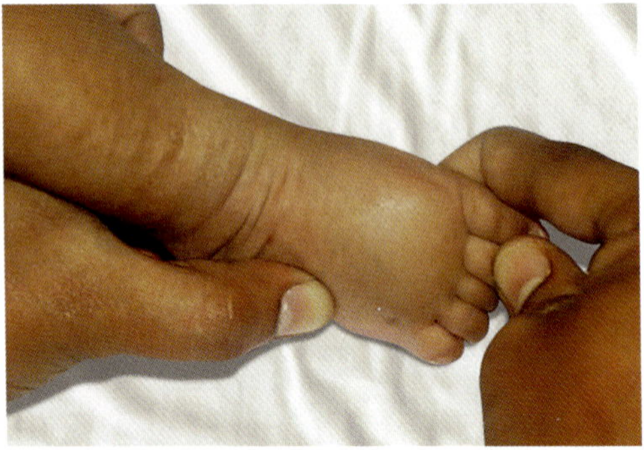

FIG. 12.3B: Clinical picture showing applying pressure at calcaneo-cuboid joint

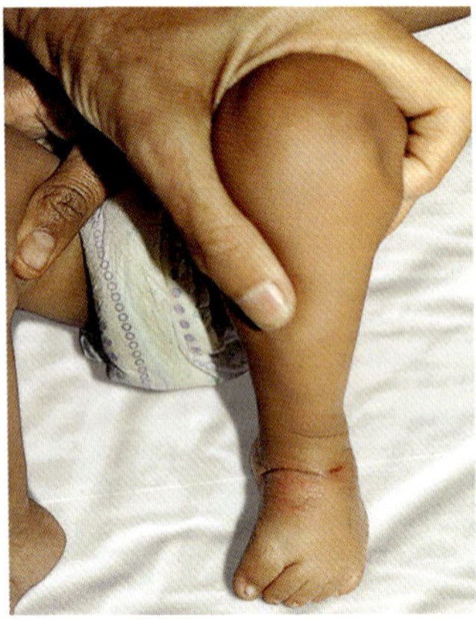

FIG. 12.4: Failed to obtain full abduction

4. *Failure to obtain full abduction of the foot*: Full abduction to 60° is necessary to reduce the talonavicular joint for correction of adduction and heel varus. Therefore, inability to correct adduction deformity increases the chances of relapse **(Fig. 12.4)**.

5. *Frequent manipulation not followed by proper immobilisation*: The foot should be immobilised in well-fitting cast with the contracted ligaments at maximum stretch after manipulation. In the cast, ligament's loosening occurs which allows more stretching at the next session. If the correction is done after cast applied it can cause folding up or wrinkling up of the cast, which can cause pressure sores **(Fig. 12.5)**.
6. *Application of below-knee instead of above-knee cast*: Above-knee plaster cast is needed to prevent the ankle and talus from rotating. As the foot must be held in abduction under the talus, the talus must not rotate, otherwise the correction obtained by manipulation will be of no use **(Fig. 12.6)**.
7. *Correction of equinus before correction of heel varus and supination*: This leads to midfoot break resulting

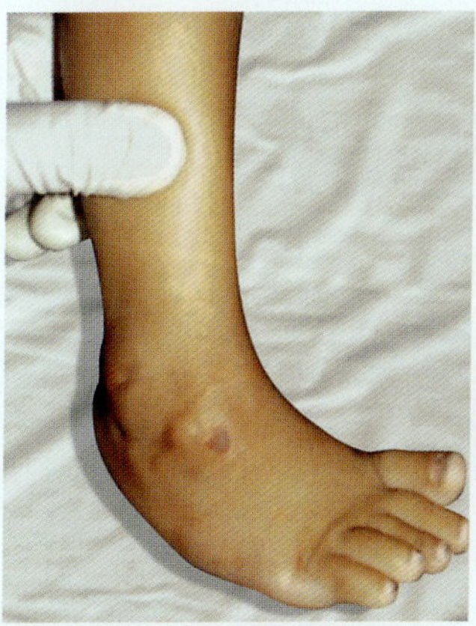

FIG. 12.5: Pressure sore at talus due to pressure after pop hardened

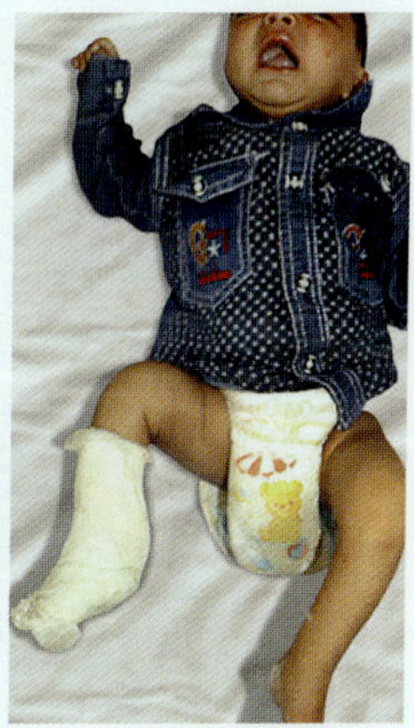

FIG. 12.6: Below knee cast

in rocker bottom deformity of foot. These problems have been avoided if fully abduct (50–60°) foot before dorsiflexion or tenotomy to make dorsiflexion easier **(Fig. 12.7)**.

8. *Attempt to obtain perfect anatomical correction*: It is wrong to assume that early alignment of the displaced skeletal elements will result in normal anatomy. Therefore, one should not overexpect to avoid overenthusiastic manipulation.
9. *Failure to use night brace*: Failure to use shoes attached to a bar in external rotation full time for 3 months and at night for 2–4 years is the most common cause of recurrence.
10. *Poor casting technique:* If too much padding is used or not enough moulding is done, then child foot can slip up inside the cast and the deformity can worsen. It is

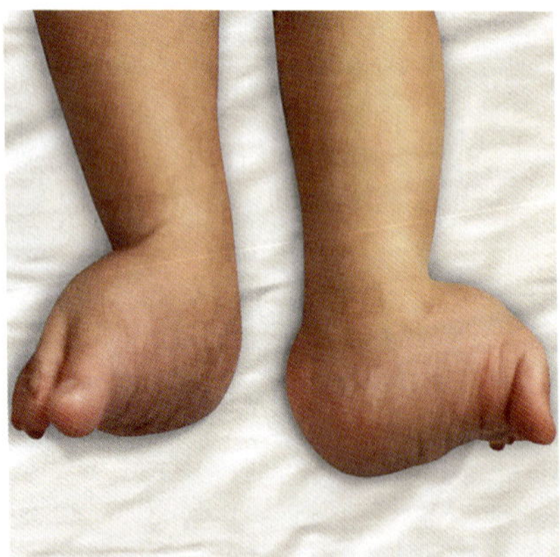

FIG. 12.7: Clinical picture of Rocker—Bottom foot due to early equinus manipulation

important to use thin layer of padding and to make the casts well fitting. Also, parents should be told to come back immediately if the foot disappears inside the cast. In the picture below, the feet slipped up inside the cast and cannot be seen. The cast is no longer doing its job and may be making the foot worse **(Fig. 12.8)**.

11. *Injecting too much local anaesthetic solution:* This can make palpation of tendon difficult and to do tenotomy **(Fig. 12.9)**.
12. *Performing a tenotomy that is too low:* The incision in the picture below is too low and can risk damage to calcaneum. Make the tenotomy at 1.0–1.5 cm above the insertion of the tendo Achilles **(Fig. 12.10)**.
13. *Incomplete tenotomy:* There should be a "pop" or "snap" as the tendon gives way, and the foot should immediately move into dorsiflexion. If this does

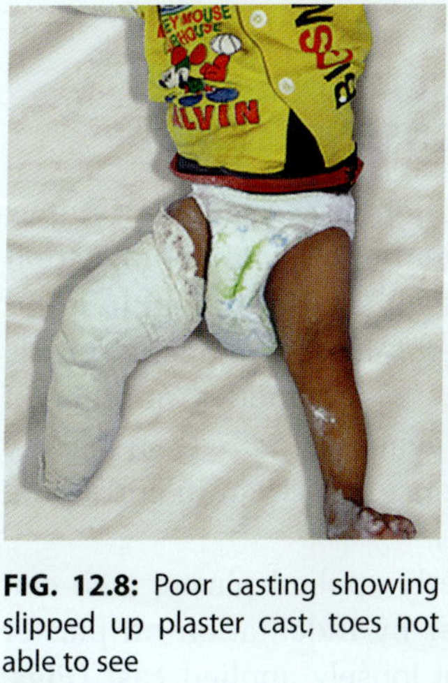

FIG. 12.8: Poor casting showing slipped up plaster cast, toes not able to see

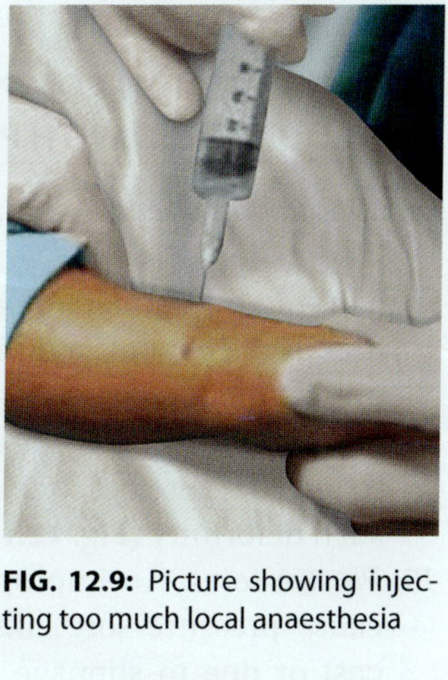

FIG. 12.9: Picture showing injecting too much local anaesthesia

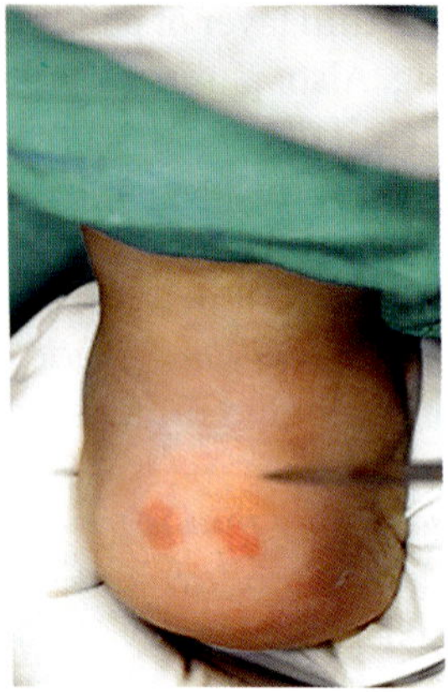

FIG. 12.10: Too low tenotomy

not happen, then it is likely that the tendon was not properly divided and you should consider repeating the procedure, if necessary.

MOST COMMON COMPLICATIONS ENCOUNTERED WITH PONSETI TECHNIQUE

14. *Metatarsal fracture due to forced correction*: Manipulation should always be gentle to avoid complication like fracture of metatarsals. It should be kept in mind that force is not required rather the technique is important for correction. In stiff foot, a number of plaster casts required are generally more than usually required, therefore, one must be patient in correcting such deformity **(Fig. 12.11)**.
15. *Plaster sores*: An improperly applied plaster cast can cause pressure sore either by indentation on plaster cast or due to slippage of loosely applied cast **(Figs. 12.12A to C)**.

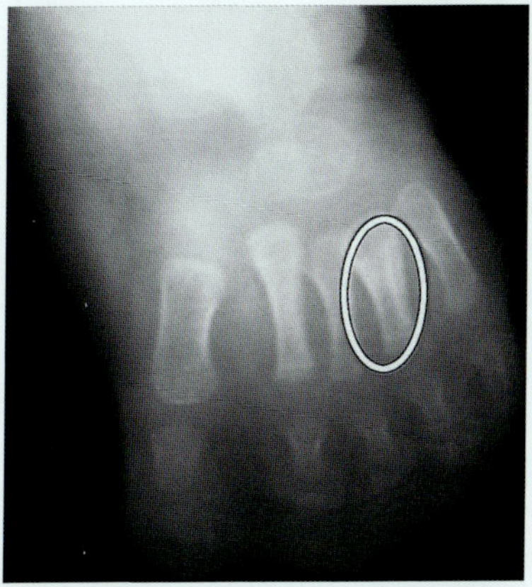

FIG. 12.11: Radiograph showing periosteal reaction after healing of metatarsal fracture due to forced correction

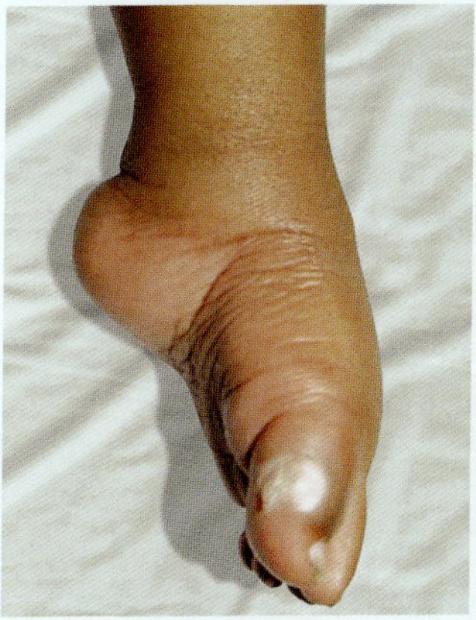

FIG. 12.12A: Plaster sore over dorsomedial aspect of great toe

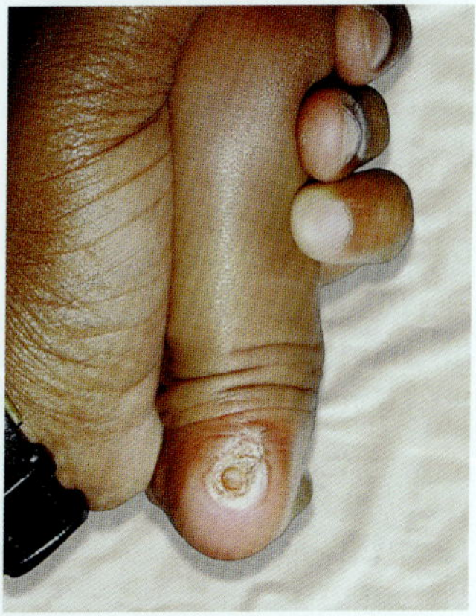

FIG. 12.12B: Plaster sore over the heel

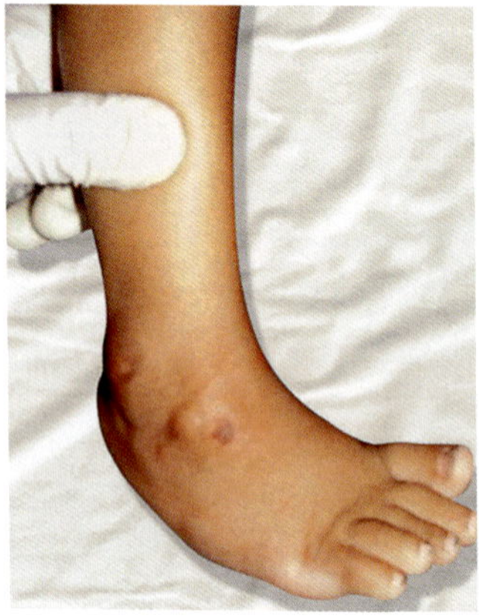

FIG. 12.12C: Plaster sore over the talar head

The nine "Clubfoot Key Messages" are described below.

1. Assess, plan, and treat
2. Talk to parents from the start (especially about braces)
3. Correct first, then maintain
4. Correct cavus first
5. Never touch the heel
6. Two people to cast
7. Toe to groin casts
8. In most cases, tenotomy is needed
9. Cover the "Talus" before the tenotomy

CHAPTER 13

Atypical Clubfoot

INTRODUCTION: ATYPICAL CLUBFOOT

Congenital idiopathic clubfoot is a deformity typically occurring in an otherwise healthy child. The most recent reports using the Ponseti method showed excellent corrections in the majority of patients. Most clubfeet correct with four to six manipulations followed by plaster cast applications by skillful orthopaedists. However, a small percentage of clubfeet are very severe and difficult to treat. They have been called very severe, stiff, and teratogenic. Numerous surgeons have performed complete, plantar, lateral, medial, and posterior releases with poor results. Relapses have been frequent.

There are a small number of clubfeet refractory to the usual corrective manipulation and casting as Turco observed. He said they "respond altogether differently to both operative and nonoperative treatment and that early surgery results in a grotesquely deformed foot." He called these feet atypical and warned against surgery.

AETIOLOGY

- Exact cause of this variant is still in debate.

- Peroneal nerve dysfunction is considered as one of the factors responsible for this variant. (This should not be confused with that of peroneal nerve palsy due to prolonged immobilisation by plaster cast in typical clubfoot, because of compression around fibular neck. In the earliest cases, the results were not fruitful whereas one can expect good results in prolonged plaster cast cases.)
- *Iatrogenic:* Slipping of typical idiopathic clubfoot in a plaster cast is an iatrogenic cause of atypical clubfoot. This slipping of cast leads to forced forefoot plantar flexion relative to the midfoot, resulting in severe midfoot cavus. It also compresses posterior calf muscles and in same process it may compress the peroneal nerve producing neurological dysfunction.

PATHOANATOMY

There may be severe involvement of gastrosoleus muscle in calf and intrinsic muscles and ligaments of sole when compared to typical clubfoot.

Calf muscles are short and Tendo-Achilles is long, wide, and very tight, pulling the calcaneus upwards leading to severe equinus and causing a deep crease above the heel. The forefoot is in adduction and all the metatarsals are in plantar flexion, causing a severe cavus and a deep crease across the sole of the foot. Although the forefoot adduction can be corrected easily with one or two plaster casts, the metatarsals remain in severe plantar flexion. Additional attempts to correct the hindfoot varus by abducting the foot deformity pushes the metatarsals and toes into additional flexion and abduction resulting in a grotesque deformity.

We suspect the abnormalities affecting the calf muscles and the posterior ligaments of the ankle extend to the deep intrinsic plantar muscles and ligaments of the foot. If the deformity is recognised as such it can be corrected with modified Ponseti technique.

CLINICAL FEATURES OF ATYPICAL CLUBFOOT

- Rigid equinus (tight Tendo-Achilles and fibrotic up to middle of the calf) **(Fig. 13.1)**
- Deep posterior crease above the heel **(Fig. 13.2)**
- Short and stubby fat feet **(Fig. 13.3)**
- Deep transverse crease present over the sole of foot **(Fig. 13.4)**
- Forefoot in adduction **(Fig. 13.5)**
- Severe supination **(Fig. 13.6)**

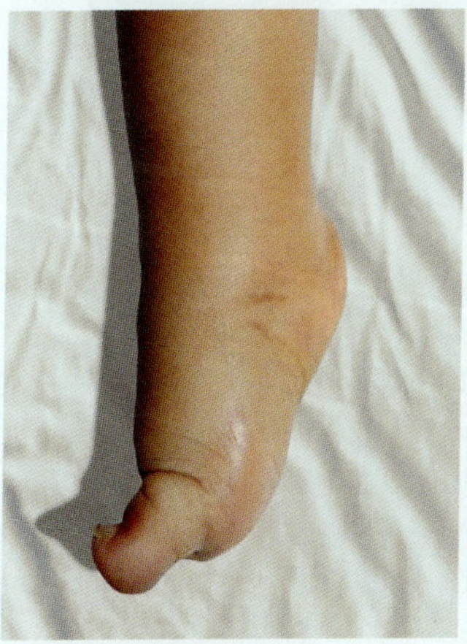

FIG. 13.1: Rigid equinus

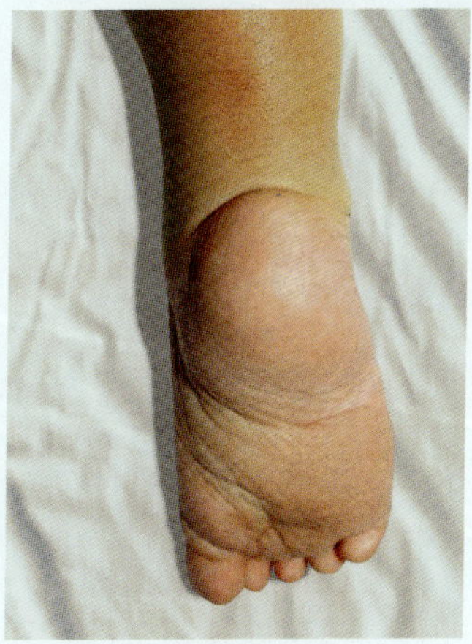

FIG. 13.2: Deep postcrease over the heel

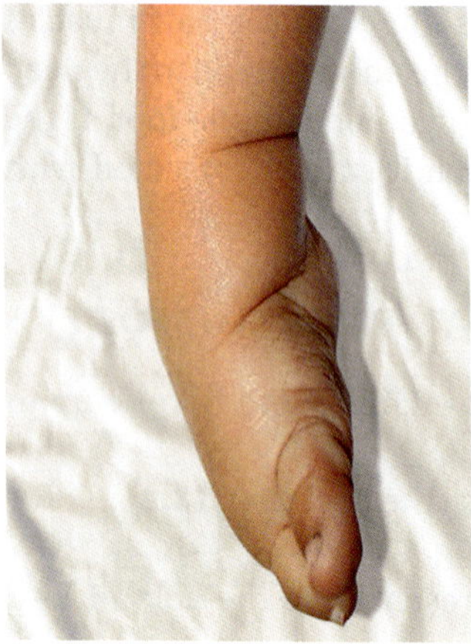

FIG. 13.3: Short and stubby foot

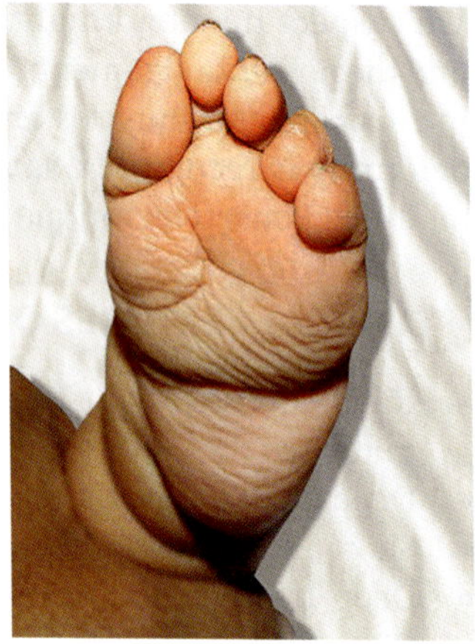

FIG. 13.4: Deep transverse crease in midfoot

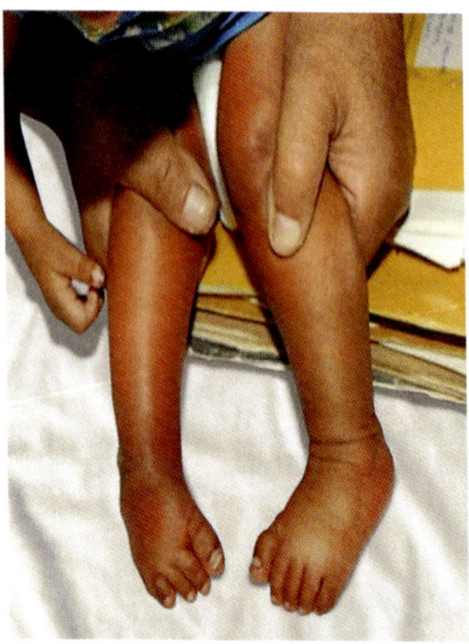

FIG. 13.5: Foot in adduction

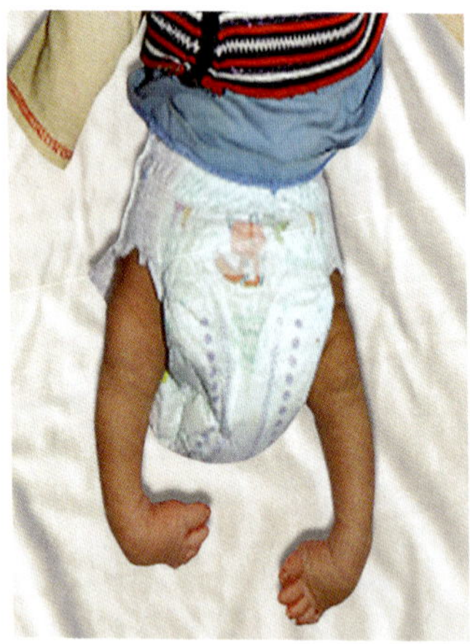

FIG. 13.6: Foot in supination

- All metatarsals were in plantar flexion, making the foot look short and arched downwards **(Fig. 13.7)**.
- Short and hyperextended first toe **(Fig. 13.8)**
- Bowing of tibia **(Fig. 13.9)**
- Lateral malleolus is always prominent.
- The calcaneus is in 50–70° of plantar flexion.
- The anterior tuberosity of the calcaneus is prominent dorsally and in contact with a small, barely identifiable head of the talus.
- The navicular is in contact with the medial malleolus.
- There is minimal motion in the severely supinated tarsal joints.
- The gastrosoleus is small and bunched up in the upper third of the leg.
- The tendo-Achillis is long and wide, inserting into the severely plantar flexed calcaneus.

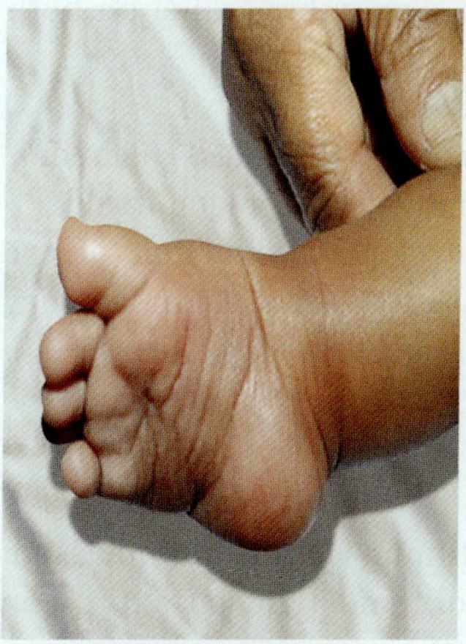

FIG. 13.7: Flexed metatarsals

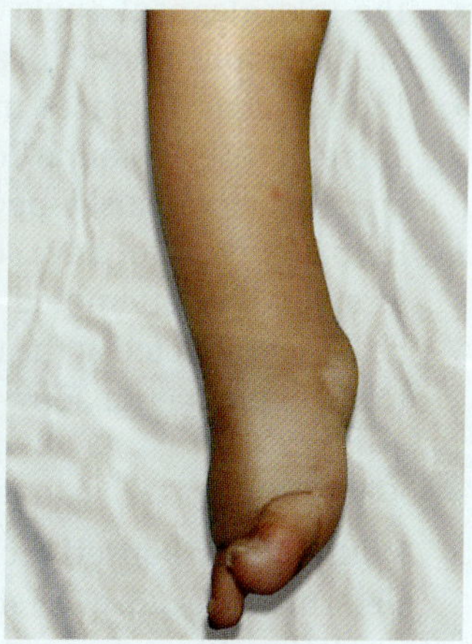

FIG. 13.8: Short and hyperextended big toe

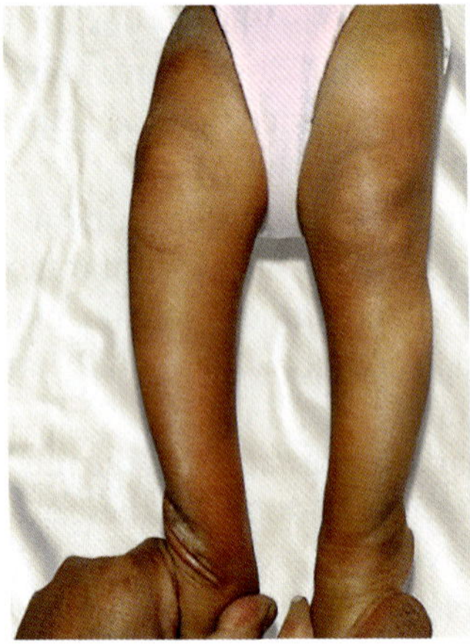

FIG. 13.9: Bowing of tibia

RADIOGRAPHIC EVALUATION (FIGS. 13.10A TO D)

- The talocalcaneal angle is generally parallel on both the anteroposterior (AP) and lateral views.
- The cuboid is displaced medially.
- There is severe plantarflexion of the talus, calcaneus, and all metatarsals, especially the first metatarsal.
- In patients who have developed abduction of the forefoot after attempted casting, the metatarsals may be hyperabducted at the tarsometatarsal joints with up to 90° of plantar flexion.

Treatment

- With regular Ponseti technique it leads to unpleasant deformity because of short and tight structures on medial and posterior aspect.
- Therefore, Ponseti proposed a modified manipulation technique and treatment protocol for this deformity.

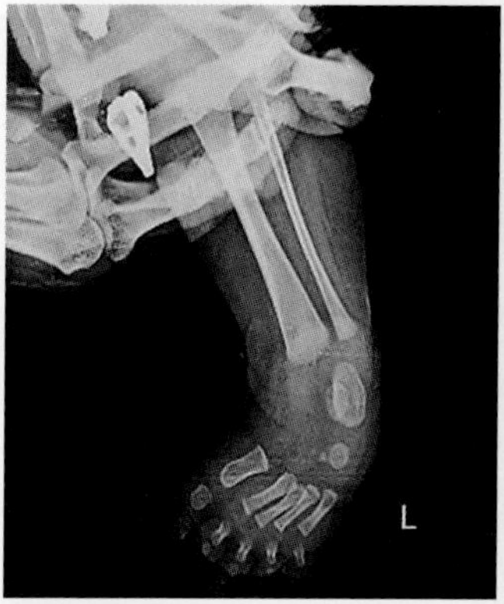

FIG. 13.10A: Atypical clubfoot 0° talocalcaneal angle

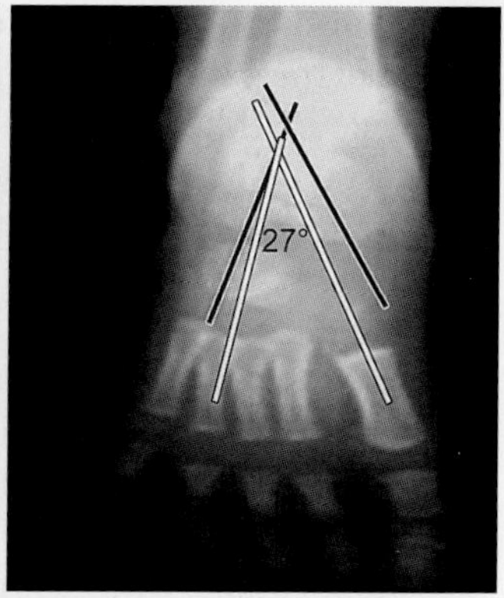

FIG. 13.10B: Normal foot 27°

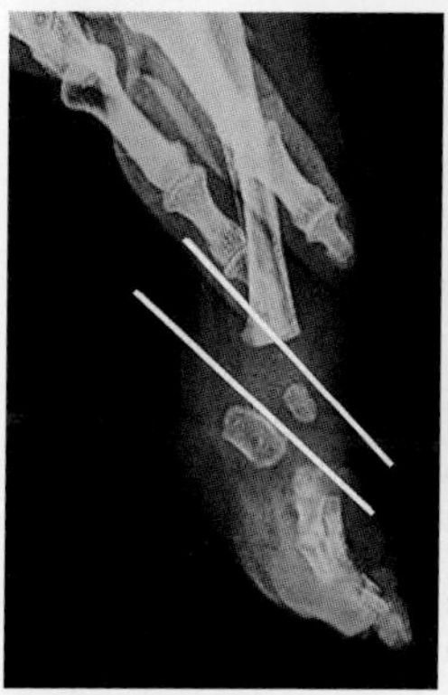

FIG. 13.10C: Atypical clubfoot 0° talocalcaneal angle in lateral view, metatarsals in plantar flexion

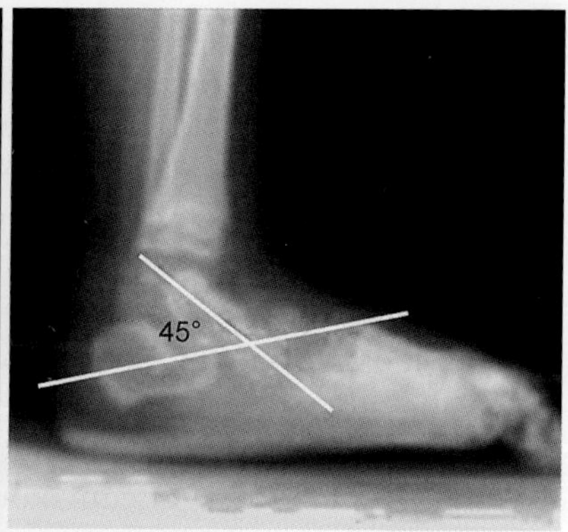

FIG. 13.10D: Normal foot 45° talocalcaneal angle in lateral view

Radiographs showing parallel talocalcaneal angle and plantar flexion of metatarsals ***(Figs. 13.10C and D)***.

What details are needed before treatment?

- Age of the patient at the first visit
- Previous treatment and type of treatment before referral
- Number of plaster casts
- Previous tendo-Achilles tenotomy or lengthening procedure.
- Correction of the deformity components
- Degree of ankle dorsiflexion after tenotomy
- Need for a second percutaneous tendo-Achilles tenotomy.
- Complications with casting
- Compliance with the foot abduction brace (assessed based on parent's reports)

Modified Ponseti Technique

- Identification of subtalar joint is required prior to the correction of the deformity. The forefoot has to be grasped with one hand while feeling the malleoli from front with the thumb and index finger of the other hand. The thumb and index finger then were moved forward to clasp the head of the talus and feel the navicular on one side and the anterior tuberosity of the calcaneus on the other side. Motion at the subtalar joint could be felt when the foot was slowly abducted and anterior tuberosity of the calcaneum moved laterally under the head of the talus. In these complex atypical clubfeet, movement at subtalar joint was minimal at first but could be felt after completion of second or third plaster cast.
- Correction also requires clear identification of talus head, which is difficult to locate because it is less prominent than anterior tuberosity of calcaneum.

To make certain of the position of the talar head during stretching and while applying the cotton and plaster cast bandage over the foot, the index finger should rest over the posterior aspect of the lateral malleolus while the thumb of the same hand applies counterpressure over the lateral aspect of the head of the talus, not on the very prominent tuberosity of the calcaneum.

- Standard abduction of 70° should not be done in atypical clubfoot. Up to 20–40° of the abduction should be done. Abduction beyond 40° leads to abduction at tarsometatarsal joints and thus disruption of this joint.
- While abduction is being done, the foot usually comes into alignment with the long axis of the leg. This usually leads to slippage of cast which may cause foot edema and skin excoriation. To prevent this the cast has to be applied with knee flexion up to 110°.
- Proper moulding of the cast was also performed. To prevent bunching of excessive cast behind the knee, we applied slab of cast anteriorly on the knee to strengthen the cast. A similar slab was applied behind ankle.
- When desired abduction was obtained, the metatarsals were still severely plantar flexed. Here another modification was performed. Thumbs of both hands were placed under the heads of 1st and 5th metatarsals. Index fingers of both hands were placed dorsally over the talar head and dorsiflexion of metatarsals and ankle was performed **(Figs. 13.11A and B)**.
- Tenotomy should be performed in all cases at 1.5 cm above the posterior deep crease. Post-tenotomy dorsiflexion of 5–10° was usually obtained. Post-tenotomy cast was applied for 3 weeks. If ankle dorsiflexion of <5° was obtained post-tenotomy then plaster cast was applied for 1 week only and a new cast was applied

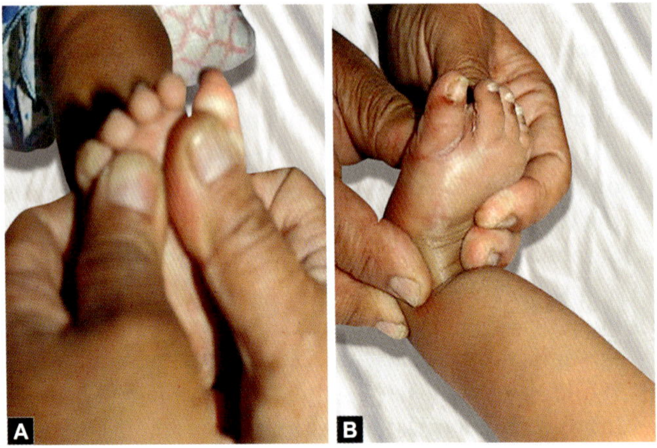

FIGS. 13.11A AND B: Pictures showing how to manipulate plantar flexion of forefoot

weekly with increasing dorsiflexion till 5–10° of dorsiflexion.

- Following cast removal, well-moulded shoes attached in 40° outer rotation to a foot abduction bar are indispensable to prevent relapses in short and stubby complex clubfeet. Brace is applied for 23 hours for first 3 months.
- During the hour when the brace was removed, two exercises were performed. One, the child was made to squat for 10 minutes. Second, the parent passively dorsiflexes the affected foot for 10 minutes.
- Following initial 3 months in brace, weaning from brace was done with 2 hours of bracing time reduced every month until night-time bracing (12 hours) was started and is advised to be kept for 3–4 years.

CASE STUDIES

Case 1

A boy aged 17 weeks was having a typical clubfoot. There was rigid equinus, severe planter flexion of all metatarsal, short hyperextended first toe, deep crease above the heel, and transverse crease in the sole of the foot. As a result, the foot is very short and stubby **(Figs. 13.12A to E)**.

Six plaster casts were applied by modified Ponseti technique. 40° abduction was achieved. Percutaneous Achillis tenotomy was performed. All the deformities were corrected. Ponseti abduction shoes were given **(Figs. 13.12F to K)**.

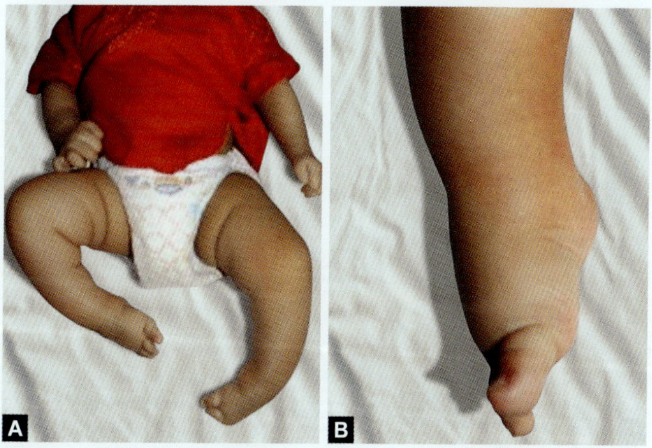

FIGS. 13.12A TO E: *Continued*

Continued

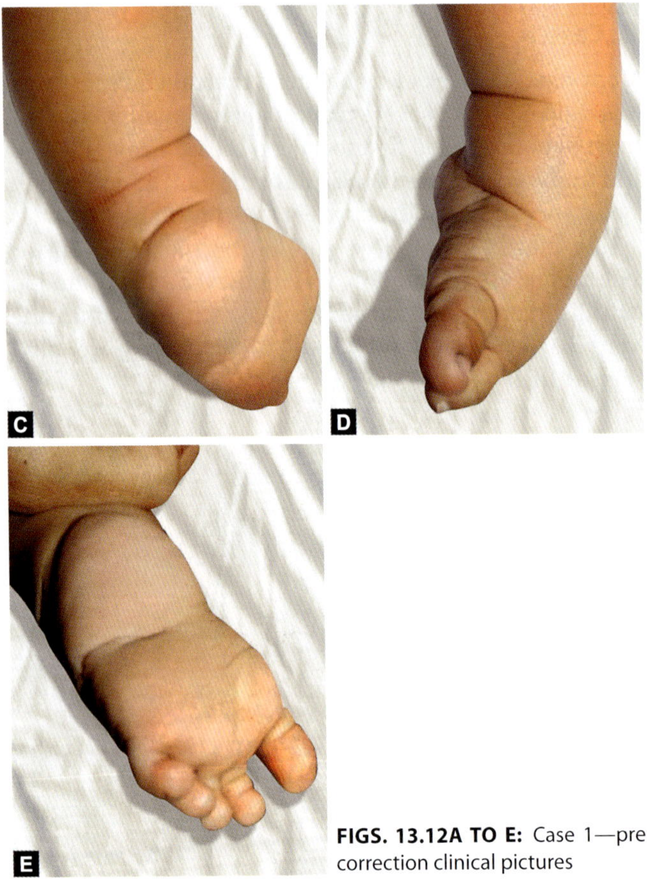

FIGS. 13.12A TO E: Case 1—pre-correction clinical pictures

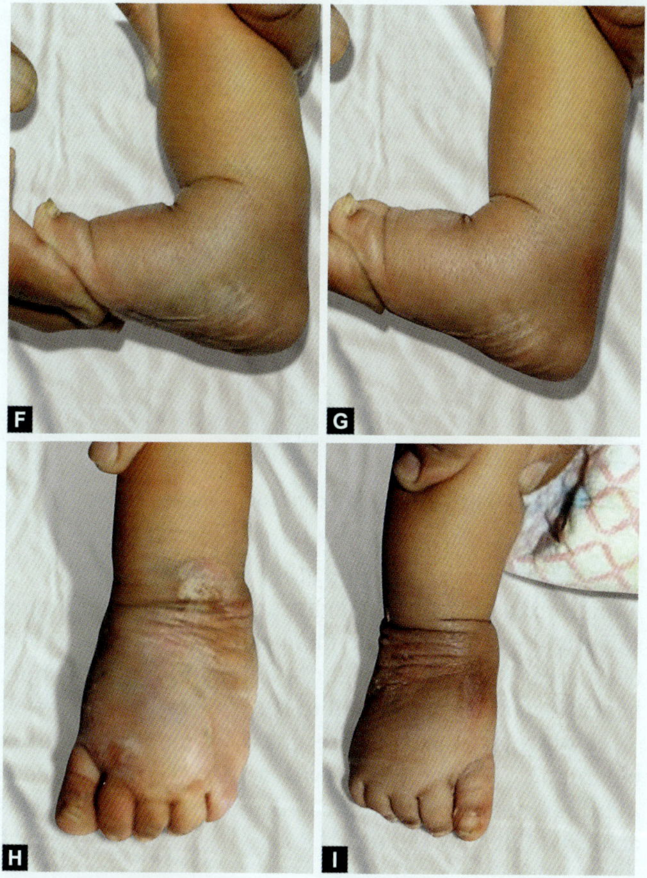

FIGS. 13.12F TO K: *Continued*

Continued

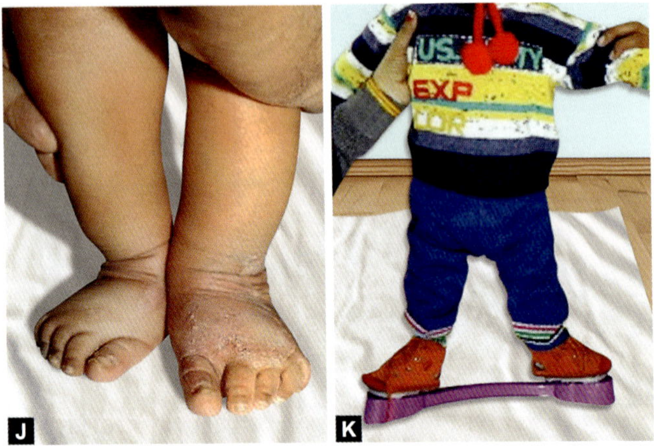

FIGS. 13.12F TO K: Case 1—post correction clinical pictures

Case 2

A male child of 13 weeks having atypical clubfoot on right side, rigid equinus, all the metatarsals in planter flexion, deep crease above the heel, the forefoot is in adduction, heel is in varus **(Figs. 13.13A to D).**

Seven plaster casts were given by modified Ponseti technique. 30° abduction was achieved. Percutaneous Achillis tenotomy was performed and plantigrade foot was achieved **(Figs. 13.13E to H)**.

Case 3

A 3-week-old male child having bilateral atypical clubfoot, rigid equinus, severe planter flexion of all metatarsal, deep crease above the heel, transverse crease in the sole of the foot, heels are in varus, and the forefoots are in adduction **(Figs. 13.14A to G)**.

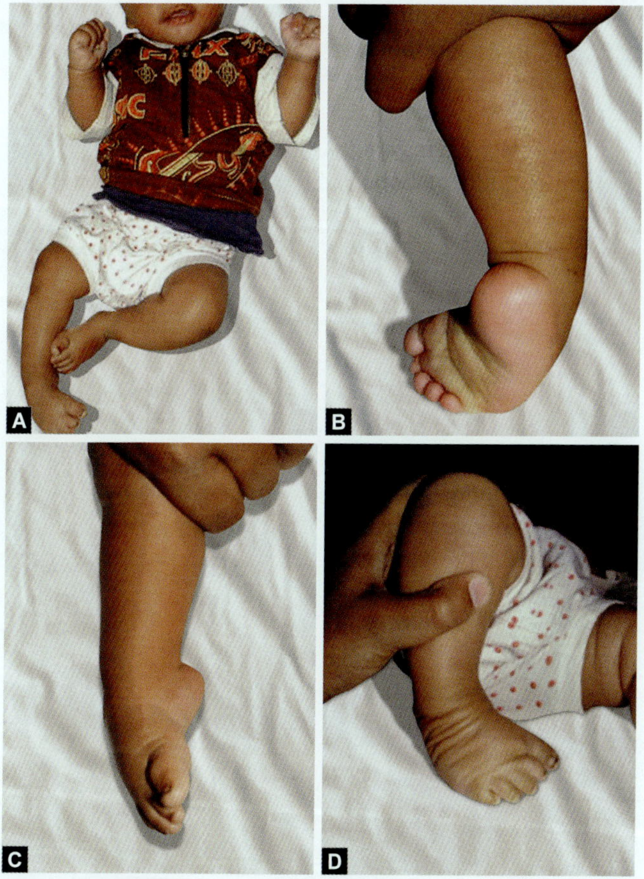

FIGS. 13.13A TO D: Precorrective photographs

Six plaster casts were applied by modified Ponseti technique. The deformities were corrected after the percutaneous Achillis tenotomy. Plantigrade foot was achieved **(Figs. 13.14H to K)**.

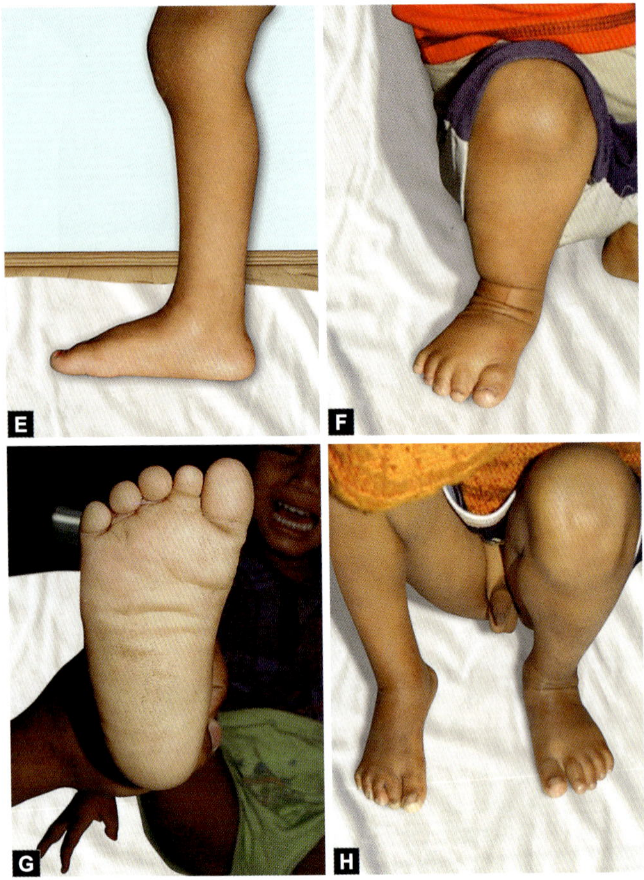

FIGS. 13.13E TO H: Case 2—post correction clinical photographs

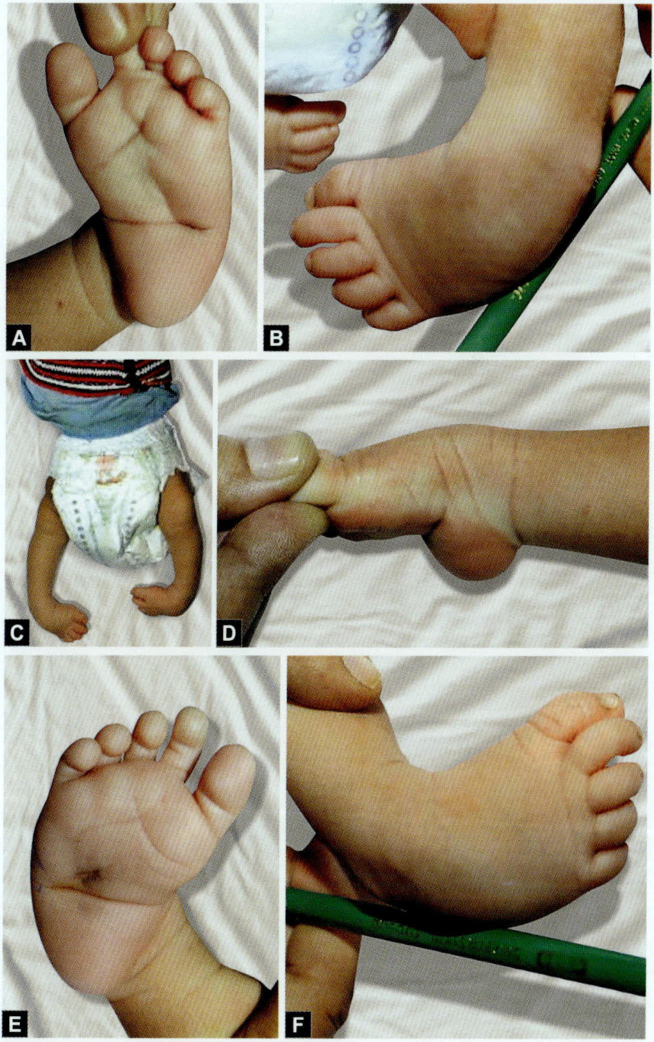

FIGS. 13.14A TO G: *Continued*

Continued

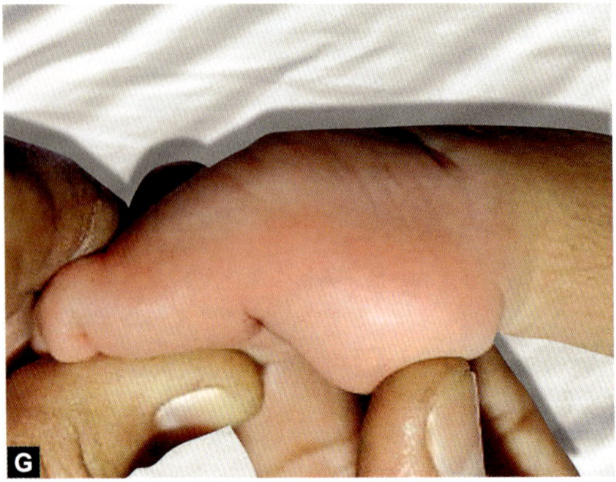

FIGS. 13.14A TO G: Case 3—bilateral precorrection clinical photographs

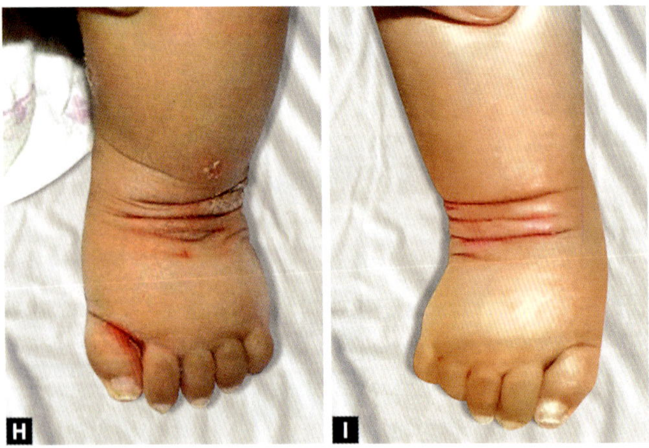

FIGS. 13.14H TO K: *Continued*

Continued

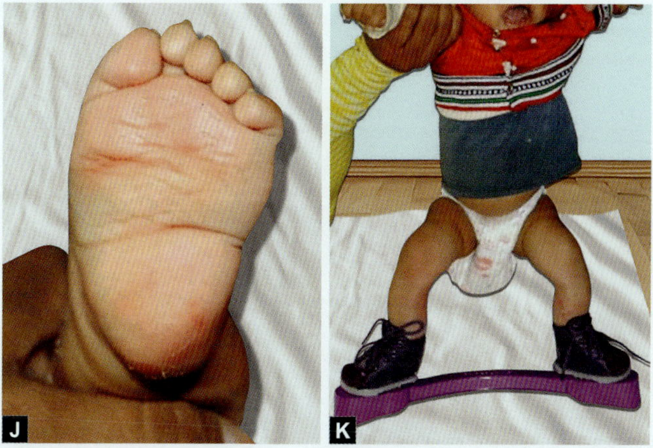

FIGS. 13.14H TO K: Case 3—bilateral post correction clinical photographs

Index

Page numbers followed by *f* refer to figure.

A

B

C

D

E

F